Peritoneal Dialysis in the Modern Era

Edited by Ayman Karkar

Published in London, United Kingdom

Peritoneal Dialysis in the Modern Era
http://dx.doi.org/10.5772/intechopen.1003481
Edited by Ayman Karkar

Contributors
Abigael Francis, Alejandro Treviño-Becerra, Ali Jasim Al Saedi, Atmane Seba, Axler Jean Paul, Ayman Karkar, Carlos Enrique Mendez-Landa, Dalia Mahmood Ali, Dalila Boumendil, Djamila Djahida Batouche, Djilali Batouche, Dulce Paola Grajales-García, Fabiola Pazos-Pérez, Fatima Souhila Bouchama, Giovanni Palleschi, Gustavo Adolfo Bautista Carbajal, Jesús Iván Lara-Prado, José Alfredo Feria-Ramírez, Karla Castillo Carpinteyro, Nariman Fahmi Ahmed Azat, Nydia Karen Cruz Escutia, Ratnadeep Biswas, Salah-eddine Benfarhi, Sam Henderson, Souad Chelghoum, Valeria Rossi, Yasir Fathi Sharba, Yessica Lopez Cabrera, Zakaria-Zoheir Addou

First published in London, United Kingdom, 2025 by IntechOpen
IntechOpen is the global imprint of INTECHOPEN LIMITED, registered in England and Wales, registration number: 11086078, 167-169 Great Portland Street, London, W1W 5PF, United Kingdom

For EU product safety concerns: IN TECH d.o.o., Prolaz Marije Krucifikse Kozulić 3, 51000 Rijeka, Croatia, info@intechopen.com or visit our website at intechopen.com.

British Library Cataloguing-in-Publication Data
A catalogue record for this book is available from the British Library

Peritoneal Dialysis in the Modern Era
Edited by Ayman Karkar
p. cm.
Print ISBN 978-1-83634-095-9
Online ISBN 978-1-83634-094-2
eBook (PDF) ISBN 978-1-83634-096-6

Meet the editor

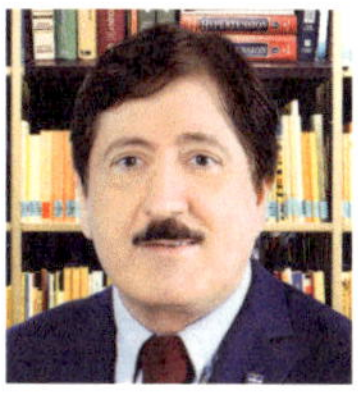

Dr. Karkar is a consultant physician, a nephrologist and a Fellow of the Royal Colleges of Physicians (FRCP) of the United Kingdom (London, Edinburgh, Glasgow, and Ireland), the American National Kidney Foundation and the American Society of Nephrology. Following graduation from medical school, Dr. Karkar received his MSc in Nephology and Hypertension and Ph.D. in Renal Medicine from the Hammersmith Hospital at the University of London in the United Kingdom. Dr. Karkar has been a Consultant Physician and Nephrologist at the Kanoo Kidney Centre (KKC), Dammam Medical Complex (DMC), Ministry of Health (MoH), Saudi Arabia from 2001- 2014. He served as director of KKC and DMC, supervising renal services in the Eastern Province of Saudi Arabia. He has served as a key advisor to the Saudi MoH and a chairman and a member of numerous steering committees, where he provided valuable assistance to the Saudi MoH, especially in setting up the dialysis outsourcing project. Dr. Karkar has a great interest in clinical research and has published around 100 papers in peer-reviewed medical/renal journals, 7 chapters, and edited 5 books in renal medicine, as well as 61 abstract publications at international conferences in nephrology. Dr Karkar has also organized and participated, as a speaker and/or chairperson, in many local and international congresses and symposia.
Dr. Karkar has a great interest in hemodialysis, peritoneal dialysis and continuous renal replacement therapies. He has contributed to the education and training of undergraduate and postgraduate medical students and nursing staff. In particular, he created theoretical and practical training courses in renal medicine. These include "Diploma in Hemodialysis", Peritoneal Dialysis" and "Continuous Renal Replacement Therapy" courses. In addition, he developed a peritoneal dialysis training program for nurses and physicians, which was commanded and accredited by the European Dialysis Transplantation Nurses Association (EDTNA). Dr. Karkar currently serves as the Head of Medical Affairs for the Middle East and Africa at the Baxter Healthcare Scientific Office.

Contents

Preface

Peritoneal dialysis is a well-established home-based kidney replacement therapy for patients with end-stage kidney disease, offering patients more lifestyle flexibility. Peritoneal dialysis has multiple benefits over hemodialysis, which include clinical, economic, and social benefits. In the past 20 years, peritoneal dialysis has witnessed significant improvements in different aspects, including pre-dialysis care and shared decision-making, glucose-sparing strategies, connecting system, improved techniques of peritoneal dialysis catheter insertion, peritoneal dialysis solutions, and cyclers with remote patient monitoring and management. Despite these valuable benefits and improvements, its global penetration rate remains low at about 12%. This is due to multiple medical and non-medical factors. Notably, the lack of awareness or inadequate patient education and implementation of shared decision-making, inadequate training of healthcare professionals, physician bias, and lack of incentives and/or reimbursement remain major impactful factors.

This book, *Peritoneal Dialysis in the Modern Era*, represents an update on selected and most important theoretical and practical aspects of peritoneal dialysis therapy, which is elegantly written by distinguished and experienced authors. Each chapter provides a clear description in a simple and easily understood layout, which is supported by illustrations and/or figures or tables. This book aims to increase awareness and update healthcare professionals on what has changed in PD practice over the past 20 years. It also provides readers with a reference to support their day-to-day clinical practice, aiming to improve the clinical outcomes of PD-treated patients.

Finally, my special thanks to the Publishing Process Manager, Ms. Maja Bozicevic, for her outstanding efforts in collecting and editing the manuscripts and her professional secretarial support.

Ayman Karkar
Consultant Physician and Nephrologist,
Baxter Scientific Office,
Head of Medical Affairs for the Middle East and Africa,
Renal Care,
Dubai, United Arab Emirates

Chapter 1

Introductory Chapter: Modern Peritoneal Dialysis

Ayman Karkar

1. Background

Peritoneal dialysis (PD) is a well-established home-based kidney replacement therapy for patients with end-stage kidney disease (ESKD), offering patients more convenience and flexibility of lifestyle. PD is empowered with an efficient natural filter or dialyzer (peritoneal membrane). Peritoneal membrane is composed of two layers (parietal and visceral) with a cavity in-between (peritoneal cavity). It is a semi-permeable membrane, rich in blood supply, and has a large surface area (1.5–2.0 m^2). The peritoneal membrane (peritoneal dialysis) allows for the exchange of solutes and fluid between the peritoneal capillary blood and the dialysis solution in the peritoneal cavity [1]. PD is based on the physiological principles of diffusion, convection, and osmosis. The removal of retained uremic toxins and excess fluid is achieved by infusing osmotic agent (like glucose) and/or colloidal solution (like icodextrin) into peritoneal cavity [2]. The infused PD solutions, which vary in volumes from 0.5–3.0 liters (depending on the age and body surface area), are introduced and removed from the peritoneal cavity through a permanent indwelling peritoneal (Tenckhoff) catheter. The PD catheter can be inserted at bedside under local anesthesia, surgically by laparoscopic technique, or by open surgical procedure. PD can either be performed manually (continuous ambulatory PD or CAPD) during the daytime or using a machine/cycler (automated PD or APD) overnight. PD prescription is achieved by performing a number of exchanges of PD solutions [3].

2. Benefits of peritoneal dialysis

Peritoneal dialysis, as a home-based therapy, has multiple benefits over those of hemodialysis (HD). These include (1) clinical benefits such as (a) preservation of residual kidney function, (b) preservation of vascular access, especially central venous catheters, (c) lower risk of infection (e.g., blood born viruses), (d) lower risk of cerebrovascular accident (no heparin is needed), (e) better early survival rate, (f) same or lower risk of mortality, (g) better bridge to kidney transplantation, (h) remote patient monitoring and management (RPM), and (i) valuable protection during pandemics (e.g., COVID-19), (2) economic benefits such as (a) more favorable hospitalization profile, (b) lower use of injectable medications, such erythropoietin stimulating agents, and (c) better employment, and (3) social benefits such as (a) self-care with positive impact on health outcomes, (b) improved patient satisfaction, and (c) better cognitive functions and quality of life [4–9].

 IntechOpen

3. Prevalence of peritoneal dialysis

Despite these benefits, the global penetration rate does not exceed 12%, though its variable among different countries [10]. Countries who pursued "PD First" policy, where PD is used as the first treatment modality for appropriate ESKD patients, as in Hong Kong who achieved high penetration rates (71%). Other countries pursued "PD Preferred", where government policy on dialysis encourages the use of PD as the treatment choice while removing any existing disincentives. These countries include China, India, Taiwan, Spain, North America, and Mexico. Alternatively, countries like Australia/New Zealand and Finland pursued "Home Dialysis First," where PD or home HD is used as the first treatment modality, usually as a complimentary strategy [11].

The low global PD penetration is due to multiple medical and non-medical factors. The absolute medical contraindications for PD are multiple adhesions with small intraperitoneal compartments, uncorrectable mechanical defects like urinary bladder exstrophy, and irreparable hernia. In addition, there are relative contraindications, which include morbid obesity, presence of ostomy, active diverticulitis, large abdominal aortic aneurysm, and severe cognitive or physical impairment [12, 13]. The non-medical reasons include lack of awareness or inadequate patient education and implementation of shared decision making (SDM), patient and/or caregiver unable or unwilling to perform the therapy, physician bias (lack or inadequate education, training or experience), and lack of incentives and/or reimbursement [14–16].

4. Peritoneal dialysis in the modern era

The era of modern PD has witnessed significant improvement in the past 20 years. These improvements include (a) implementation of shared and informed decision-making by patients in selecting the preferred dialysis modality [17, 18], (b) pre-dialysis education and training for potential PD patients [19–21], (c) advanced laparoscopic techniques for PD catheter insertion [22], (d) glucose sparing strategies [23–25], (e) monitoring and managing PD patients remotely [26, 27], especially during pandemics like COVOD-19 [28, 29], and (f) unplanned urgent start programs [30, 31]. Furthermore, the international clinical guidelines (e.g., International Society of PD and KDIGO guidelines) have largely contributed to improved PD clinical outcomes, including technique survival and time-on-therapy. These achievements in the era of modern PD, when compared to HD therapy, resulted in lower mortality rate during the early years on dialysis [reviewed in 4], similar long-term survival rate including patients with controlled diabetes [32], improved technique [26] and patient's survival, reduced rate of adverse events (e.g., metabolic and fluid overload) and hospitalization by RPM [27], better cognitive functions and quality of life, and lower rates of post kidney transplantation delayed graft dysfunction [reviewed in 4].

Author details

Ayman Karkar
Baxter Scientific Office, Medical Affairs, Dubai, United Arab Emirates

*Address all correspondence to: han94dan97@gmail.com

References

[1] Choi P, Brown EA. Peritoneal dialysis. Medicine. 2003;**31**(6):70-73. DOI: 10.1383/medc.31.6.70.28314

[2] Ellam T, Wilkie M. Peritoneal dialysis. Medicine. 2015;**43**(8):484-488. DOI: 10.1016/j.mpmed.2015.05.001

[3] Teitelbaum I, Burkart J. Core curriculum in nephrology: Peritoneal dialysis. American Journal of Kidney Diseases. 2003;**42**(5):1082-1096. DOI: 10.1053/S0272-6386(03)01123-5

[4] Karkar A, Wilkie M. Peritoneal dialysis in the modern era. Peritoneal Dialysis International. 2023;**43**(4):301-314. DOI: 10.1177/08968608221114211

[5] Agarwal S, Wilkie M. Peritoneal dialysis. Medicine. 2023;**51**(3):209-214. DOI: 10.1016/j.mpmed.2022.12.011

[6] Lambie M, Davies S. An update on absolute and relative indications for dialysis treatment modalities. Clinical Kidney Journal. 2023;**16**(Suppl. 1):i39-i47. DOI: 10.1093/ckj/sfad062

[7] François K, Bargman JM. Evaluating the benefits of home-based peritoneal dialysis. International Journal of Nephrology and Renovascular Disease. 2014;**7**:447-455. DOI: 10.2147/IJNRD.S50527

[8] Gamage I, Dhar A, Tregaskis P, Wilson S. Frequency and risk factors for cognitive dysfunction in peritoneal dialysis patients. Nature Reviews Nephrology. 2022;**27**(12):945-952. DOI: 10.1111/nep.14117

[9] Raoofi S, Kan FP, Hoseinipalangi Z, Rezaei S, Ahmadi S, Masoumi M, et al. Hemodialysis and peritoneal dialysis-health-related quality of life: Systematic review plus meta-analysis. BMJ Supportive and Palliative Care. 2023;**13**(4):365-373. DOI: 10.1136/bmjspcare-2021-003182

[10] USRDS 2024 Annual Data Report. International Comparisons – 2022 Data. End Stage Renal Disease: Chapter 11. Available from: https://usrds-adr.niddk.nih.gov/2024/end-stage-renal-disease/1-incidence-prevalence-patient-characteristics-and-treatment-modalities [Accessed: March 2025]

[11] Liu FX, Gao X, Inglese G, Chuengsaman P, Pecoits-Filho R, Yu A. A global overview of the impact of peritoneal dialysis first or favored policies: An opinion. Peritoneal Dialysis International. 2015;**35**(4):406-420. DOI: 10.3747/pdi.2013.00204

[12] Blake PG, Quinn RR, Oliver MJ. Peritoneal dialysis and the process of modality selection. Peritoneal Dialysis International. 2013;**33**(3):233-241. DOI: 10.3747/pdi.2012.00119

[13] Teitelbaum I. Peritoneal dialysis. The New England Journal of Medicine. 2021;**385**(19):1786-1795. DOI: 10.1056/NEJMra2100152

[14] Li PKT, Chow KM, Van de Luijtgaarden MWM, Johnson DW, Jager KJ, Mehrotra R, et al. Changes in the worldwide epidemiology of peritoneal dialysis. Nature Reviews Nephrology. 2017;**13**:90-103. DOI: 10.1038/nrneph.2016.181

[15] Manns B, Agar JWM, Biyani M, Blake PG, Cass A, Culleton B, et al. Can economic incentives increase the use of home dialysis? Nephrology Dialysis Transplantation. 2019;**34**(5):731-741. DOI: 10.1093/ndt/gfy223

[16] Sloan CE, Coffman CJ, Sanders LL, Maciejewski ML, Lee SYD, Hirth RA, et al. Trends in peritoneal dialysis use in the United States after Medicare payment reform. Clinical Journal of the American Society of Nephrology. 2019;**14**(12):1763-1772. DOI: 10.2215/CJN.05910519

[17] Blake PG, Brown EA. Person-centered peritoneal dialysis prescription and the role of shared decision-making. Peritoneal Dialysis International. 2020;**40**(3):302-309. DOI: 10.1177/0896860819893803

[18] Brown EA, Blake PG, Boudville N, Davies S, de Arteaga J, Dong J. International society for peritoneal dialysis practice recommendations: Prescribing high-quality goal-directed peritoneal dialysis. Peritoneal Dialysis International. 2020;**40**(3):244-253. DOI: 10.1177/0896860819895364

[19] Karkar A. The value of pre-dialysis care. Saudi Journal of Kidney Diseases and Transplantation. 2011;**22**(3):419-427

[20] Van den Bosch J, Warren DS, Rutherford PA. Review of predialysis education programs: A need for standardization. Patient Prefer Adherence. Dove Press. 2015;**9**:1279-1291. DOI: 10.2147/PPA.S81284

[21] Heaf J, Heiro M, Petersons A, Vernere B, Povlsen JV, Sørensen AB, et al. First-year mortality in incident dialysis patients: Results of the peridialysis study. BMC Nephrology. 2022;**23**:229. DOI: 10.1186/s12882-022-02852-1

[22] Shrestha BM, Shrestha D, Kumar A, Shrestha A, Boyes SA, Wilkie ME. Advanced laparoscopic peritoneal dialysis catheter insertion: Systematic review and meta-analysis. Peritoneal Dialysis International. 2018;**38**(3):163-171. DOI: 10.3747/pdi.2017.00230

[23] Holmes C, Mujais S. Glucose sparing in peritoneal dialysis: Implications and metrics. Kidney International. 2006;**70**:S104-S109. DOI: 10.1038/sj.ki.5001924

[24] PKT L, Culleton BF, Ariza A, Do JY JDW, Sanabria M, Shockley TR, et al. Randomized, controlled trial of glucose-sparing peritoneal dialysis in diabetic patients. Journal of the American Society of Nephrology. 2013;**24**(11):1889-1900. DOI: 10.1681/ASN.2012100987

[25] Bonomini M, Zammit V, Divino-Filho JC, Davies SJ, Di Liberato L, Arduino Arduini A, et al. The osmo-metabolic approach: A novel and tantalizing glucose-sparing strategy in peritoneal dialysis. Journal of Nephrology. 2020;**34**(2):503-519. DOI: 10.1007/s40620-020-00804-2

[26] Corzo L, Wilkie M, Vesga JI, Lindholm B, Buitrago G, Rivera AS, et al. Technique failure in remote patient monitoring program in patients undergoing automated peritoneal dialysis: A retrospective cohort study. Peritoneal Dialysis International. 2022;**42**(3):288-296. DOI: 10.1177/0896860820982223

[27] Paniagua R, Alfonso Ramos A, Ávila M, MDJ V, Nevarez-Sida A, Qureshi A, et al. Remote monitoring of automated peritoneal dialysis reduces mortality, adverse events and hospitalizations: A cluster-randomized controlled trial. Nephrology, Dialysis, Transplantation. 2025;**40**:588-597. DOI: 10.1093/ndt/gfae188

[28] Brown EA, Perl J. Increasing peritoneal dialysis use in response to the COVID-19 pandemic: Will it go viral? JASN. 2020;**31**:1928-1930. DOI: 10.1681/ASN.2020050729

[29] Bunch A, Ardila F, Castaño R, Quiñonez S, Corzo L. Through the

storm: Automated peritoneal dialysis with remote patient monitoring during COVID-19 pandemic. Blood Purification. 2021;**50**:279-282. DOI: 10.1159/000511407

[30] Jin H, Fang W, Wang L, Zang X, Deng Y, Wu G, et al. A randomized controlled trial comparing automated peritoneal dialysis and hemodialysis for urgent-start dialysis in ESRD. Kidney International Reports. 2024;**9**:2627-2634. DOI: 10.1016/j.ekir.2024.06.032

[31] Lee JY, Cho H, Park JH, YI. Comparison of survival outcomes in haemodialysis versus immediate-start peritoneal dialysis: A propensity-matched study. Nephrology. 2025;**30**(1):e14418. DOI: 10.1111/nep.14418

[32] Elsayed ME, Morris AD, Li X, Browne LD, Stack AG. Propensity score matched mortality comparisons of peritoneal and in-centre haemodialysis: Systematic review and meta-analysis. Nephrology, Dialysis, Transplantation. 2020;**35**(12):2172-2182. DOI: 10.1093/ndt/gfz278

Chapter 2

Quality of Life in Patients Undergoing Peritoneal Dialysis

Giovanni Palleschi and Valeria Rossi

Abstract

In the last years, various manuscripts suggest that patients undergoing peritoneal dialysis have better quality of life than those submitted to hemodialysis. While studies in the past were limited by poor cohorts and the use of non-validated methods, more recently the literature has provided better data from meta-analyses and systematic reviews. In various studies, the quality of life of patients undergoing dialysis is lower than that of healthy subjects and is burdened either by symptoms related to chronic disease or by disadvantages that are associated with treatments. This burden becomes worse in subjects receiving replacement therapies. Even if comparative data are not unanimous, there is a tendency in favour of peritoneal dialysis with respect to haemodialysis regarding physical status, mental status, the general perception of health and tolerability versus treatment. Patients undergoing peritoneal dialysis usually report better autonomy, lower anxiety, a good relationship with the medical staff and lower pain when compared to subjects receiving haemodialysis. However, a higher statistical difference between peritoneal dialysis and hemodialysis in terms of quality of life is achieved only about the general impact of kidney disease, and some of the recent studies still report non-definitive conclusions. This report summarizes the current evidence on the topic.

Keywords: chronic renal failure, peritoneal dialysis, quality of life, health-related quality of life, burden, end-stage renal disease

1. Introduction

The World Health Organization defines Quality of Life (QOL) as an individual's perception of their position in life in the context of the culture and value systems in which they live and in relation to their goals, expectations, standards and concerns [1]. Quality of life represents an indicator of the state of health of patients especially in those suffering from chronic diseases, because it also helps to obtain information about disease evolution. The aim of diagnostic and therapeutic interventions is not only to eradicate pathologic conditions but also to restore adequate QOL, providing patients with health, which is considered a "state of complete physical, mental and social well-being and not merely the absence of disease and infermity" [2]. Poor QOL is often associated with chronic pathologic conditions and multimorbidity, being disease severity, duration, and patterns of symptoms as the most influencing factors [2, 3]. Understanding the impact that a specific disease determines on patients' QOL is of utmost importance to assess at the best how people deal with a pathological condition and which measures can be adopted to improve their status [4]. This aspect is better known as "Health related Qol (HRQOL)", defined as "health aspects of QOL, generally considered to reflect the impact of disease and treatment on disability and daily functioning" [4]. As with many other chronic disorders, chronic kidney disease (CKD) negatively affects QOL and patients who need replacement therapies (dialysis) report poorer perceived health [5]. The assessment of QOL in people suffering from CKD has been the object of investigation for many years, and a large amount of data is available from the literature. However, the studies often differ in patients' numbers, methods of investigation, statistical assessment and parameters considered. A significant rate of manuscripts specifically describes outcomes of QOL in CKD patients undergoing replacement therapies, haemodialysis (HD) and peritoneal dialysis (PD). Some of these studies present comparative data between the two dialytic techniques, while some others are focused only on the outcomes of one type of treatment. The aim of this chapter is to summarize the more recent data about QOL in patients undergoing PD and also to explore outcomes when compared with subjects undergoing HD.

2. Research strategy

Both the authors G.P. and V.R. independently performed research on the topic through the database PubMed using the following keywords: chronic renal failure, peritoneal dialysis, quality of life, health-related quality of life, burden, and end-stage renal disease. We considered feasible for our investigation the manuscripts published in literature since the last 10 years, to provide quite recent evidence on the argument. We examined only papers published in English starting from the systematic reviews and meta-analyses, then choosing the studies with a larger number of patients and preferring those that adopted similar, standardized and validated tools for QOL assessment. Additional references with older publication dates, and considered of interest for the purpose of this research, were then extracted from the lists and citations of the manuscripts reviewed. Metanalyses and systematic reviews reporting comparative data on QOL between PD and HD were also included in the investigation. We aimed to describe the most significant outcomes reported by literature about the impact of PD on the lives of patients in order to provide a state of the art of current knowledge on this important field of research.

3. Quality of life in patients undergoing peritoneal dialysis

3.1 Prevalence of PD

Peritoneal dialysis represents one method of kidney replacement therapy. Epidemiological data and quite recent surveys report that it accounts for about 9–15% of treatments in patients suffering from end-stage renal disease (ESRD) in the world [6]. Data provided by the International Society of Nephrology Global Kidney Health Atlas (ISN-GKHA) in 2018 indicate that PD median global prevalence is about 38.1 per million population, with significant differences among countries because this type of therapy is not worldwide available [7]. In fact, this survey reports that in 2018 PD was not utilized in 30 countries, especially in low-income ones in Africa [7]. However, this scenario is probably going to change in the future years: some advantages of PD compared to HD, such as higher feasibility, easier management, good cost-effectiveness ratio, could contribute to implementing the use of this type of replacement therapy in many countries [7]. Therefore, while in the US and Europe HD still covers a larger rate of replacement therapies, in the Middle East and Asian regions a higher use of PD is registered; Hong Kong has been reported as the place with the highest use of PD in the world [8].

3.2 Assessment and standardization of quality of life in PD patients

Among replacement therapies available for the treatment of ESRD, a major rate of patients undergo HD and for this reason, the surveys performed on subjects submitted to PD exploring QOL and psychological issues, especially in the past, have been unpowered by poor populations [9]. However, it has been reported that this is often the consequence of the lack of specific methods of investigation and standardized instruments to assess how QOL is burdened by PD [10]. Therefore, standardizing and prioritizing PD outcomes, including QOL assessment, has become a goal of clinicians, researchers and Scientific Societies [10, 11]. The International Society for Peritoneal Dialysis (ISPD) has promoted research to provide a standardization of PD outcomes developing validated methods for the procedure and prompting the use of well-recognized tools for QOL assessment [11]. This programme is intended to overcome the limits in QOL assessment when based only on clinicians' evaluation and diagnosis [10]. Very recently, standardized definitions of PD-related symptoms and complications have been described including clinical criteria for a correct diagnosis, and have been reported by literature [11]. Various systematic reviews and metanalyses reporting PD outcomes focused on symptoms and complications usually sub-divide data into different categories: pain, gastro-intestinal symptoms, fatigue, depression, anxiety, muscular symptoms (cramps), pruritus, restless legs syndrome, sexual function, sleep disorders [10]. All these symptoms may be responsible for QOL worsening because of social, mental and physical disability, reduction of life participation and carer burden [5, 9]. Some of these disturbances can be a direct consequence of PD treatment, while some others are also sustained by the pathophysiological mechanisms of ESRD, especially as the consequence of fluid volume status, blood pressure changes, mineral and bone disorders, anemia [9, 12]. It is not always easy to distinguish whether the impact on the patient's QOL is more related to the chronic disease or to dialysis treatment and it is for this reason that many studies compare PD with HD, in order to prevent a possible incorrect interpretation of the results. In addition, the studies that provide high-quality data are those that adopted dedicated instruments (questionnaires) for QOL assessment [11]. Patient Report Outcomes (PRO) represent, in fact, the best tools to assess patients' perceptions because directly reporting patients' feelings. In studies assessing PRO in subjects undergoing PD the following questionnaires were the most used: Short-Form Health Survey 36 (SF-36), (Euro Quality of Life—5D), Kidney Disease Quality of Life (KDQOL), MOS social support survey, MMSE (Mini Mental Scale Examination) [10]. All these questionnaires have been submitted to specific processes to be recognized as valid and reliable and are widely used in clinical trials.

3.3 Comparing the quality of life in PD vs. HD patients

3.3.1 The impact of PD on patients' physical and mental status and effects of social support on the quality of life

Many studies suggest that PD diminishes the QOL of patients if compared with healthy subjects and that during years of treatment, the QOL scores tend to worsen due to a perception of both physical and mental health deterioration [9]. This outcome is common in almost all patients suffering from chronic pathologic disorders [3]. In addition, patients undergoing dialysis, including those submitted to PD, show to lose personal hope during the time, as the replacement therapy prolongs and a chance of relief or receiving a kidney transplant reduces [12]. This outcome is strongly correlated to the impairment of functional status (one of the strongest predictors of all PROs), that is negatively conditioned by dialytic therapy that limits daily activities [12]. Although data from the literature show that PD globally lowers QOL scores, the studies highlight somewhat differences among countries because social support, availability of expert caregivers and economic resources are not the same everywhere [7, 13]. In fact, as confirmed by large surveys, social support appears to be a "key factor" considering the perception of QOL. Sitjar-Suner et al. 2020 conducted research with the purpose of assessing HRQOL and perceived social support in patients undergoing PD [5]. The authors performed a cross-sectional multicenter investigation from 2015 to 2017 to assess feelings experienced by patients undergoing PD in real life using the KDQOL and the MOS social support [5]. The population was represented mostly by men, with at least 5 years of dialytic age. The results showed a significant impact of PD on patients' emotional status, social interaction, sleep, general perception of health, mental status and sexual activity, being this last aspect reported more by men than women (with prevalence reaching 64% of the population) and especially represented by erectile dysfunction [5, 14–16]. Specifically, regarding treatment, a large number of patients reported satisfaction and good relationships with the staff, but they confirmed that PD caused limitations on their daily activities, and life participation, inducing most of them to make adaptations in their lives and in the lives of the family [6, 14]. A subgroup with a severe reduction in QOL was represented by people who declared that they could not work after starting to receive PD. Furthermore, a significant rate of patients described personal difficulty in sharing feelings and experiences of dialysis with other people [5]. One important variable that was significantly associated with negative perception in QOL was hospitalization. On the other side, all patients who reported receiving good and effective social support were those with better scores in QOL. As an additional outcome, this study showed that people with previous experience with HD described PD as less aggressive and better tolerated. Many investigations report that PD is well tolerated by patients; studies with an observational time longer than the research of Suner [5] reveal that physical and mental status may improve in some patients during the time, generally after 24 months of treatment [17]. This outcome is usually different in patients undergoing HD, who in some studies perceive a deterioration of social interaction, and physical and mental status [18]. Mental status has a crucial role in HRQOL, because anxiety, and loss of hope, often associated with a negative psychological condition, can lead to depression which is described as an important issue also in PD patients although still underestimated [9, 12, 19, 20]. One of the most important aspects that appear to determine a deterioration in QOL and depression in patients undergoing dialysis is pain [20]. Pain may be generally the consequence of some pathophysiological mechanisms of CKD, in particular bone mineral disorders, but it can be also influenced by the dialytic technique and could require adjustment of dialysate composition [21–23]. Davison et al. in 2005 reported that pain was independently related to depression and sleep disorders in patients undergoing dialysis [21]. Moreover, other authors have shown that the severity of pain in subjects undergoing dialysis is associated with vascular and other tissue calcification, that are consequent to parathyroid hormone alterations (causing bone pain), with consequent negative impact on physical component, mental component scale, negatively influencing global PD outcomes [22–26]. Among the most important aspects that resulted to be affected by pain, in fact, there are physical activity and the quality of sleep [27–29]. The great attention that literature has focused on pain is definitely justified by the fact that this symptom is the most important factor that contributes to affect QOL [6]. A detailed analysis of the incidence of pain in patients submitted to PD has been performed by Chunyan et al. in 2022 [30]. This research included a large cohort, consisting of 463 patients submitted to PD, whose perception of pain was investigated by means of the Short-Form Mc Gill Pain Questionnaire (SF-MPQ). The prevalence of pain in this population is 33.1%. The outcomes supported that pain was associated mostly with bone and mineral disorders, considering that normal levels of calcium, phosphorus and parathyroid hormone were poorly associated with symptoms. Statistical analysis has shown older age and elevated parathyroid hormone levels to be risk factors for developing pain in PD patients of this cohort. The most interesting finding was that patients with higher scores regarding pain perception were those with poorer QOL also because they needed to assume analgesics, confirming that many of them suffered from sleep disturbances that were associated with anxiety and depression. Being the consequence of pain and other conditions, sleep disorders are prevalent in the PD population (ranging from 69 to 81%), and are often associated with fatigue and depression with a negative effects on QOL [27, 28]. Principal aspects of QOL in PD patients and here reported are represented in **Table 1**.

List of items	Outcome
Social interaction and life participation	Not uniformly assessed by studies [10]—Treatment may limit participation in various activities [14]—Patients report needing adaptations in their lives due to dialytic treatment and sharing their experience is difficult [5].
Pain	This symptom may be initially present but can improve over time [21]—Pain is usually associated with infusion and drainage of dialytic solutions [23] and may be the consequence of bone metabolism disorders, with negative mental and physical impact [21, 23, 24, 29].
Physical status/ fatigue	It is associated with age [31, 32], female sex [31, 32], higher BMI [31], unemployment and low physical activity [31, 33]. Fatigue contributes to reducing social interaction [17]—Patients can report perceiving less energy and less strength with consequent emotional distress [5, 34].
Mental status and depression	Prevalence ranges between 28 and 40% and it is underestimated [13]—It is associated with low functional status and it has a negative impact on QOL [13, 20]—PD patients describe that ignorance and misunderstanding by people of their condition had negative consequences on their mental status [5].
Sexual dysfunction	The condition is prevalent in PD patients, reaching 64% in large cohorts, and mostly represented by erectile dysfunction in men, with a negative impact on QOL [14–16].
Sleep	Studies adopting proper methods, such as the *Pittsburgh Slee Quality Index,* report prevalence between 69 and 81% [27, 28]—Sleep disturbances are associated with fatigue, depression, and reduced QOL [27, 35]—Many patients doing treatment at home during nighttime report that this can interfere with rest and sleep [5, 14].

Patients outcomes regarding the main aspects that influence QOL in subjects receiving PD are reported.

Table 1.
Principal aspects of quality of life in PD patients.

3.3.2 Comparative outcomes on quality of life of PD and HD patients from systematic reviews and metanalysis

As above mentioned, much data regarding QOL in PD patients comes from studies that compare outcomes of HD with those of PD. Generally, comparative investigations describe higher benefits on patients' QOL from PD than HD, although some data are still controversial [18]. The results of the most important surveys on QOL in PD patients are summarized by systematic reviews and meta-analysis. A schematic representation of the main outcomes resumed in this paragraph is shown in **Table 2**. A very important meta-analysis performed by the group of Samira Raoofi in 2023 reported results after reviewing 147 studies comprehensive of a total number of 623,728 individuals [36]. In this work, studies using SF-36 and KDQOL short-form questionnaires were included, while researches not in English were excluded. This investigation was based on the Newcastle–Ottawa Scale for the assessment of the quality of papers, and

Authors/references	Type of study	Outcome
Raoofi et al. [36]	Meta-analysis of 147 studies including 623,728 patients	Patients undergoing PD have greater lifestyle confirmed by better scores at domains of the questionnaires regarding emotional dimension, environment, and social interactions [37]—PD patients present higher life flexibility in lifestyle [38].
Chuasuwan et al. [39]	Metanalysis on 7995 studies (finally examined 21)	PD patients had better scores regarding physical functioning [40, 41], role limitations [42], pain [43, 44], general health [44], and energy [44]. Physical functioning and role limitations were the domains with statistical significance [39].
Goncalves et al. [45]	Survey on 338 patients	QOL scores better in PD patients in work status, encouragement from dialysis staff, and satisfaction with treatment (with statistical significance). HD patients had better results in physical and emotional functioning.
Wright et al. [14]	Survey on 77 patients	PD patients had the highest QOL scores regarding physical functioning, emotional well-being, and general health (with no statistical significance).
Griva et al. [34]	Survey on 433 patients	QOL scores were better in PD patients regarding satisfaction in relation to treatment. HD and PD patients had similar scores in other domains.
Okpechi et al. [22]	Survey on 86 patients	QOL scores were better in PD patients but without statistical significance.
Kim et al. [46]	Survey on 237 patients	QOL scores were better in PD patients with statistical significance regarding the domain of symptoms list.
Wakeel et al. [47]	Survey on 200 patients	QOL scores better with statistical significance in PD patients except for physical functioning.
De Abreu et al. [48]	Survey on 350 patients	QOL scores better in PD patients regarding constant encouragement and support by dialysis staff. HD patients presented better QOL improvement at 12-month check-up.

The table shows the main results regarding QOL assessment provided by the most important studies comparing PD and HD treatment. PD patients usually present higher QOL scores; however, the difference appears statistically significant not in all the studies and not in all the domains of the questionnaires. The sub-analysis of KDQOL-SF domains shows that the impact of kidney disease is significantly lower in PD patients than in those undergoing HD.

Table 2.
Comparative outcomes of main QOL aspects between PD and HD patients based on KDQOL-SF questionnaire results. Meta-analysis and most important studies are reported.

it is described as the first worldwide systematic review and meta-analysis examining the HRQOL and the determinants across patients who underwent HD and PD. As the main result of this protocol, the authors observed in some studies greater lifestyle in PD patients with better scores in emotional, environmental and social interaction domains [37] as a consequence of higher life flexibility [38]. They also reported an inverse relationship between QOL and age, and a significant inverse relationship between age and Body Mass Index (BMI) in patients undergoing dialysis, while QOL resulted to decrease in dialytic age as reported also by other researchers [22]. Other authors report that outcomes in patients undergoing HD and PD get worse in the elderly [31, 32] and that fatigue is associated with age [29] and BMI [26, 31], reducing daily activities [30, 33]. Poor HRQOL in subjects undergoing dialysis is confirmed to be affected by several factors, such as loss of independence, loss of employment, and social life reduction, with consequent psychological negative outcomes [49]. Social limitation consequent to the dialytic treatment and fatigue appears to be the main cause leading to poor scores in QOL domains regarding physical (perception of less strength and less energy), mental and emotional status [5, 14, 32]. Furthermore, some data provide evidence that QOL in patients undergoing HD and PD proportionally decreases the deterioration of general medical condition which is often also associated with economic troubles [33]. Data specifically focused on the comparison between HD and PD outcomes from this metanalysis support the evidence that patients undergoing PD have greater lifestyle confirmed by better scores at domains of the questionnaires regarding emotional dimension [5]. The possibility to choose time for treatment, at a comfortable place, decreases the risk of anxiety and depression, even if some studies report that nocturnal PD can interfere with rest and sleep [5, 35]. In fact, despite the fact that PD patients can do the treatment at home, which should result in more comfort, in some studies, both PD and HD patients present similar rates in investigations on sleep quality [35]. A less restrictive dietary programme, higher autonomy in doing treatment and the longer preservation of residual diuresis resulted to be factors favoring better PD outcomes in comparison with HD: these aspects have been suggested by some authors as factors that reduce functional dependency of patients respect to treatment [50]. A metanalytic study designed by Chuasuwan et al. in 2020 included 7995 publications (comprehensive of abstracts from congresses) leading to a final examination of 21 papers [39]. Investigational methods were represented by SF-36, KDQOL and Eq. 5D. The outcomes showed that regarding physical functioning [40, 41, 51], role limitations [42], pain [43, 44], general health [52], the scores were significant better in PD than HD patients. However, it has been reported that the difference in the scores in the majority of sub-domains resulted not always statistically significant [50]. Specifically, using the unstandardized mean difference (USMD) of QOL between PD and HD groups, only the sub-domain scores of physical functioning and role limitations were confirmed significantly higher in PD than in HD ones. One of the main factors responsible for better QOL scores in PD patients was confirmed to be the chance to make treatment in comfortable places with respect to dialysis centres/hospitals. In 2017 Zazzeroni et al. carried out a specific metanalysis on manuscripts published from 2011 to 2016 [52]. The authors identified 946 articles but at the end of the process, they considered only seven. In the conclusions, they reported that data were not unanimous and that not all the manuscripts reported a statistically significant difference regarding QOL between the two treatments [52]. Particularly, they observed that some of the studies [14, 17] reported better scores in PD patients only in a few domains of the questionnaires (work status, support by the dialysis staff and satisfaction of the patient).

In addition, they found also manuscripts reporting better QOL and better satisfaction in HD patients when they were assessed at long follow-up, and on home treatment; these patients showed to achieve better scores in the domains regarding social interaction [14]. Other studies show better outcomes in QOL of PD than HD patients without a statistically significant difference at the sub-domain's examination, as reported by Okpechi et al. [22]. However, the cohort examined in this protocol was limited to a single renal hospital unit. Otherwise, this paper shows an interesting correlation in PD patients between good emotional condition and blood levels of ferritin and hemoglobyn concentration, while pathological levels of calcium (low concentration) and parathyroid hormone are shown to be associated with bad symptoms, such as fatigue and bone pain, especially in HD subjects [17]. Favorable outcomes in terms of global QOL, especially concerning satisfaction related to treatment, levels of anxiety and depression, were reported by other groups of PD patients [34, 45, 46]. Wright et al. in 2015 evaluated QOL in HD and PD patients during a 6 months period: HD patients on home treatment showed better outcomes than subjects undergoing in-centre HD [14]; the best favorable scores were reported by subjects treated by PD, even if also in this study the difference was not statistically significant at the sub-domain examination. An interesting experience has been reported by Badri Man Shreshta from Sheffiled, who generically described better QOL provided by PD with respect to HD because of higher autonomy, better flexibility, reduced number of hospital visits and potential longer preservation of residual kidney function and diuresis that represents a significant advantage, especially for patient's candidate for transplant [53]. This group remarks that despite significant reported advantages of PD respect HD, the first technique is underutilized especially in US and Europe, for reasons that are not completely explored and understood. Additional outcomes were provided by Wakeel in 2012 on 200 patients showing better QOL scores in PD patients except for physical functioning and by De Abreau in 2011 who reported similar outcomes in a survey on 350 individuals, especially regarding constant encouragement and support by PD staff [47, 48]; in this last study, HD patients had better QOL improvement after 12 months of treatment [47, 48].

3.3.3 Factors influencing quality of life and satisfaction level in PD patients: Pre-dialysis care, shared decision-making, assisted treatment and remote control

Various factors can influence QOL and satisfaction in patients receiving PD. The choice of treatment in patients suffering from ESRD represents a major decision, with significant consequences on their QOL. First of all, important studies show that proper pre-dialysis education and social support can increase the choice of PD by patients [54, 55]. It has been reported by various experiences that shared decision-making could play a favorable role in achieving a good QOL with treatment [56]. This process directly involves patients who receive information about replacement therapies from caregivers through the use of videos, dedicated courses and printed material [57]. While some studies have controversial outcomes, reporting that, despite detailed counseling, patients finally declared to follow clinicians' suggestions and to feel themselves with passive respect to the process of decision [54], some others demonstrated the positive impact of multi-disciplinary pre-dialysis care (MDPC) on the treatment outcomes [57]. Specifically, MDPC has been shown to improve patients' survival and to be associated with a larger rate of patients starting dialysis treatment with PD [57, 58]. I-Kuan Wang and collaborators examined the impact of multi-disciplinary pre-dialysis care (MDPC) on a large group of 672 patients undergoing PD, of those 126 subjects under the usual care and 546 under MDPC on the risk of peritonitis, technique failure and mortality [59]. The results showed that diabetic patients had a lower risk of mortality due to the MDPC. The association between earlier pre-dialysis care with higher PD choice and better patient QOL and survival has been demonstrated also by Dandara N Spigolon and collaborators in 2016, after a survey performed on 4107 patients receiving PD from 2004 and 2011 [60]. Other authors describe that a well-organized outpatient office and service capable of providing adequate information and support to patients can contribute to direct to PD, showing that in many countries the patient's orientation to HD may often be the consequence of the lack of organizational assessment and social support [61]. In the future, dedicated outpatient facilities are warranted to give patients adequate knowledge about replacement techniques allowing them to choose the treatment that can provide them with better QOL. As many authors report, in fact, shared decision-making should stand as a standard of care [61]. Another important factor that can influence the QOL of patients receiving PD is represented by the availability of assistance. Well-structured programmes contributing to improve the QOL of PD patients have been prompted in some countries by the chance to perform assisted treatment at patients' homes with several advantages and benefits [61]. An assisted PD may be necessary especially in the elderly but also in specific categories of patients that for various reasons cannot be completely autonomous [62]. Studies performed on large communities show that assisted PD is more utilized in non-academic centres [63]. With respect to the past, in the last 10 years assisted PD has increased in many countries and this improvement has positively influenced the choice of PD as replacement therapy in ESRD showing good clinical outcomes and providing satisfaction in QOL [64]. This result has allowed us to overcome various barriers that have limited in the past the use of PD especially in elderly and fragile patients [65]. However, in different scenarios, an assisted PD could not be available due to the inaccessibility of caregivers. This is the case for patients who live in rural sites that are not easy to reach due to the type of terrain, or people that live very far from medical centres. In these conditions patients could receive support by a remote control that is usually realized by data transmission through electronic devices and internet connections; furthermore, patients can be monitored by web cams that facilitate dialog and improve confidence and quality of relationship with clinicians [66, 67]. Despite literature still scarce with definitive data, the studies available show that remote control can help patient to have better management of treatment and clinicians in making decisions, leading to better care and outcomes, including QOL [65–67].

3.3.4 Considerations

Chronic Kidney Disease incidence and prevalence are increasing in the world. This condition is associated with high cardiovascular risk and it is responsible for an increased risk of death [68]. Although kidney transplant represents the best treatment for patients suffering from ESRD, a large rate of CKD patients receives replacement therapies: HD and PD. These procedures have significantly improved in the last 20 years gaining more favorable results and contributing to providing patients with better prognosis and better life expectancy. For this reason, QOL assessment has become more important in this condition because it provides information about the impact and the evolution of the disease [5]. Quality of life in patients suffering from CKD has been deeply investigated by literature showing a negative effect that involves physical and mental status [35]. Among individuals with CKD, QOL strongly deteriorates in hospitalized patients and in those receiving replacement therapies [6].

Data presented in this chapter summarize the main outcomes provided by literature in the last 10 years about QOL in patients receiving PD. The analysis of papers that we considered for this investigation supports the use of dedicated tools for QOL assessment in patients undergoing dialysis. The meta-analysis examined suggests that PD reduces the QOL of patients compared with healthy subjects, because of symptoms related to CKD and disadvantages and complications associated with treatment [5]. Furthermore, scores regarding QOL tend to worsen with dialytic age due to a reduced perception of health status. In fact, in patients receiving PD, symptoms' representation affects QOL, reducing scores of physical and mental conditions. No statistically significant difference was found among the sexes regarding the variables included in the QOL questionnaires, even if some studies reported more limitations on sexual activity described by men than women. Comparative data between PD and HD outcomes provide the most part of information regarding QOL. The prevalence of studies supports better QOL outcomes in patients receiving PD in terms of physical functioning, role limitations, pain, general health and energy. High statistical significance is reported regarding the lower impact that CKD has on PD than HD patients. Various authors describe additional factors in favor of PD that contribute to improve QOL in comparison with HD individuals: reduced number of hospital admissions, better cosmesis (due to the different body access for treatment associated with lower pain compared to repeated cannulations of artero-venous fistula in HD subjects), a higher flexibility for managing time of treatment and better autonomy. Since a larger number of researchers has prompted adequate surveillance of QOL in patients undergoing dialysis as a routinary method included in the global patients' assessment, some advantages of PD have become more evident and well recognized by literature. Several studies have also shown that at least 50% of patients candidate for replacement therapy due to ESRD prefer PD when properly informed about the two dialytic techniques available [69]. This evidence is quite in contrast with the diffusion in the world of PD, which is the less utilized dialytic technique, accounting for around 15% of all dialysis treatment in European countries and the US [70]. The underutilization of PD may recognize various causes, such as lack of training in clinicians and caregivers and factors related to the choices made by public healthcare systems that include the mechanism of financial remuneration [70, 71]. However, this aspect will surely need to be better explored by future studies that should include also economic issues.

4. Conclusions

The assessment of QOL is an undeniable part of patients' evaluation, especially in the case of chronic diseases. The outcomes of QOL contribute to a better understanding of the course of the disease and to adequately estimate the efficacy of treatment. In addition, these instruments may help healthcare systems to adequately plan strategies and resources to face the burden of disease. The large number of studies on QOL in patients undergoing PD clearly show that these subjects have poorer QOL than healthy subjects either due to a direct effect of CKD and also due to the burden associated with dialytic treatment, which lowers physical and mental conditions. However, despite some studies reporting similar and comparable QOL outcomes among the two dialytic techniques, from the majority and more recent metanalysis, the results are in favor of PD regarding the impact of CKD. In addition, PD allows the preservation of residual diuresis with consequent maintenance of the function of the urinary tract that represents conditions predisposing for a successful kidney transplant.

Author details

Giovanni Palleschi* and Valeria Rossi
Nefrocenter Dialysis Company, Frascati, Rome, Italy

*Address all correspondence to: giovanni.palleschi@santagostino.it

References

[1] Costa DSJ, Mercieca-Bebber R, Rutherford C, Tait MA, King MT. How is quality of life defined and assessed in published research? Quality of Life Research. 2021;**30**(8):2109-2121. DOI: 10.1007/s11136-021-02826-0

[2] Post MWM. Definitions of quality of life: What has happened and how to move on. Topics in Spinal Cord Injury Rehabilitation. 2014;**20**:167-180

[3] Makovski TT, Schmitz S, Zeegers MP, Stranges S, van den Akker M. Multimorbidity and quality of life: Systematic literature review and meta-analysis. Ageing Research Reviews. 2019;**53**:100903. DOI: 10.1016/j.arr.2019.04.005. Epub 2019 Apr 30

[4] Haraldstad K, Wahl A, Andenæs R, Andersen JR, Andersen MH, Beisland E, et al. A systematic review of quality of life research in medicine and health sciences. Quality of Life Research. 2019;**28**(10):2641-2650. DOI: 10.1007/s11136-019-02214-9. Epub 2019 Jun 11

[5] Sitijar-Suner M, Suner-Soler R, Masià-Plana A, Chirveches-Pèerez E, Bertran-Noguer C, Fuentes-Pumarola C. Quality of life and social support of people on peritoneal dialysis: Mixed methods research. International Journal of Environmental Research and Public Health. 2020;**17**:4240. DOI: 10.3390/ijerph17124240

[6] Mills KT, Xu Y, Zhang W, Bundy JD, Chen C-S, Kelly TN, et al. A systematic analysis of worlwide population-based data on the global burden of chronic kidney disease. Lancet. 2017;**389**:1238-1252. DOI: 10.1038/ki.2015.230

[7] Bello AK, Levin A, Lunney M, Osman MA, Ye F, Ashuntantang GE, et al. Status of care for end stage kidney disease in countries and regions worldwide: International cross sectional survey. BMJ. 2019;**367**:l5873. DOI: 10.1136/bmj.l5873

[8] Kwong VW, Li PK. Peritoneal dialysis in Asia. Kidney Diseases (Basel). 2015;**1**(3):147-156

[9] Lew SQ, Piraino B. Quality of life and psychological issues in peritoneal dialysis patients. Seminars in Dialysis. 2005;**18**(2):119-123. DOI: 10.1111/j.1525-139X.2005.18215x

[10] Bello AK, Okpechi IG, Osman MA, Cho Y, Cullis B, Htay H, et al. Epidemiology of peritoneal dialysis outcome. Nature Reviews. Nephrology. 2022;**18**(12):779-793. DOI: 10.1038/s41581-022-00623-7. [Therefore data provided by the investigations about PD principal outcomes and QOL are characterized by significant variability lo stesso BELLO AK 2022]

[11] Elphick E, Holmes M, Tabinor M, Cho Y, Nguyen T, Harris T, et al. Outcome measures for technique survival reported in peritoneal dialysis: A systematic review. Peritoneal Dialysis International. 2022;**42**(3):279-287. DOI: 10.1177/0896860821989874. Epub 2021 Apr 21

[12] Shek Nam Ng M, Kwok Wei So W, Chow Choi K, Chen J, Sze Ho Wong S, Hui YH, et al. Hope, quality of life, and psychological distress in patients on peritoneal dialysis: A cross-sectional study. Journal of Health Psychology. 2023;**28**(13):1238-1249. DOI: 10.1177/13591053231176262. Epub 2023 May 28

[13] Brown EA, Zhao J, McCullough K, Fuller DS, Figueiredo AE, Bieber B, et al.

Burden of kidney disease, health-related quality of life, and employment among patients receiving peritoneal dialysis and In-center hemodialysis: Findings from the DOPPS program. American Journal of Kidney Diseases. 2021;**78**(4):489-500.e1. DOI: 10.1053/j.ajkd.2021.02.327. Epub 2021 Apr 16

[14] Wright LS, Wilson L. Quality of life and self-efficacy in three dialysis modalities: Incenter hemodialysis, home hemodialysis, and home peritoneal dialysis. Nephrology Nursing Journal. 2015;**42**(5):463-476; quiz 477

[15] Navaneethan SD, Vecchio M, Johnson DW, Saglimbene V, Graziano G, Pellegrini F, et al. Prevalence and correlates of self-reported sexual dysfunction in CKD: A meta-analysis of observational studies. American Journal of Kidney Diseases. 2010;**56**(4):670-685. DOI: 10.1053/j.ajkd.2010.06.016

[16] Vecchio M, Navaneethan SD, Johnson DW, Lucisano G, Graziano G, Querques M, et al. Treatment options for sexual dysfunction in patients with chronic kidney disease: A systematic review of randomized controlled trials. Clinical Journal of the American Society of Nephrology. 2010;**5**(6):985-995. DOI: 10.2215/CJN.09081209. Epub 2010 May 24

[17] Manera KE, Ju A, Baumgart A, Hannan E, Qiao W, Howell M, et al. Patient-reported outcome measures for life participation in peritoneal dialysis: A systematic review. Nephrology, Dialysis, Transplantation. 2021;**36**(5):890-901. DOI: 10.1093/ndt/gfaa244

[18] Hiramatsu T, Okumura S, Asano Y, Mabuchi M, Iguchi D, Furuta S. Quality of life and emotional distress in peritoneal dialysis and hemodialysis patients. Therapeutic Apheresis and Dialysis. 2020;**24**(4):366-372. DOI: 10.1111/1744-9987.13450

[19] Boateng EA, East L. The impact of dialysis modality on quality of life: A systematic review. Journal of Renal Care. 2011;**37**(4):190-200. DOI: 10.1111/j.1755-6686.2011.00244.x

[20] Mahajan S, Tiwari SC, Kalra V, Masih JA, Bhowmik DM, Bansal R, et al. Analysis of depression and its effect on outcome among adult Indian peritoneal dialysis patients. Peritoneal Dialysis International. 2007;**27**(1):94-96

[21] Davison SN, Jhangri GS. The impact of chronic pain on depression, sleep, and the desire to withdraw from dialysis in hemodialysis patients. Journal of Pain and Symptom Management. 2005;**30**(5):465-473. DOI: 10.1016/j.jpainsymman.2005.05.013

[22] Okpechi IG, Nthite T, Swanepoel CR. Health-related quality of life in patients on hemodialysis and peritoneal dialysis. Saudi Journal of Kidney Diseases and Transplantation. 2013;**24**(3):519-526. DOI: 10.4103/1319-2442.111036

[23] Bunchman TE, Ballal SH. Treatment of inflow pain by pH adjustment of dialysate in peritoneal dialysis. Peritoneal Dialysis International. 1991;**11**(2):179-180

[24] Wang AY. Vascular and other tissue calcification in peritoneal dialysis patients. Peritoneal Dialysis International. 2009;**29**(Suppl. 2):S9-S14

[25] Eckardt KU, Kasiske BL. Kidney disease: Improving global outcomes. Nature Reviews. Nephrology. 2009;**5**(11):650-657. DOI: 10.1038/nrneph.2009.153. Epub 2009 Sep 29

[26] Elsurer R, Afsan B, Mercanoglu E. Bone pain assessment and relationship with parathyroid hormone and health related quality of life in hemodialysis. Renal Failure. 2013;**35**(5):667-672. DOI: 10.3109/0886022X.2013.780617

[27] Guney I, Atalay H, Solak Y, Altintepe L, Toy H, Tonbul HZ, et al. Predictors of sleep quality in hemodialysis patients. The International Journal of Artificial Organs. 2010;**33**(3):154-160. DOI: 10.1177/039139881003300304

[28] Buysse DJ, Reynolds CF 3rd, Monk TH, Berman SR, Kupfer DJ. The Pittsburgh sleep quality index: A new instrument for psychiatric practice and research. Psychiatry Research. 1989;**28**(2):193-213. DOI: 10.1016/0165-1781(89)90047-4

[29] Tentori F. Focus on: Physical exercise in hemodialysis patients. Journal of Nephrology. 2008;**21**(6):808-812

[30] Yi C, Ye H, Lin J, Chang Y, Zhang X, Zhou T, et al. The incidence of pain and its association with quality of life in patients with peritoneal dialysis. Renal Failure. 2022;**44**(1):724-730. DOI: 10.1080/0886022X.2022.2068444

[31] Maruyama Y, Nakayama M, Ueda A, Miyazaki M, Yokoo T. Comparison of fatigue between dialysis modalities. A cross sectional study. PLoS One. 2021;**16**:e0246890

[32] Ossareh S, Roozbeh J, Krishnan M, Liakopoulos V, Bargman JM, Oreopoulos DG. Fatigue in chronic peritoneal dialysis patients. International Urology and Nephrology. 2003;**35**(4):535-541. DOI: 10.1023/b:urol.0000025610.67447.b9. Erratum in: Int Urol Nephrol. 2004;36(3):477

[33] Bonner A, Wellard S, Caltabiano M. The impact on fatigue on daily acitivity in people with chronic kidney disease. Journal of Clinical Nursing. 2010;**19**:3006-3015

[34] Griva K, Kang AW, Yu ZL, Mooppil NK, Foo M, Chan CM, et al. Quality of life and emotional distress between patients on peritoneal dialysis versus community-based hemodialysis. Quality of Life Research. 2014;**23**(1):57-66. DOI: 10.1007/s11136-013-0431-8. Epub 2013 May 21

[35] Eryavuz N, Yuksel S, Acarturk G, Uslan I, Demir S, Demir M, et al. Comparison of sleep quality between hemodialysis and peritoneal dialysis patients. International Urology and Nephrology. 2008;**40**(3):785-791. DOI: 10.1007/s11255-008-9359-2. Epub 2008 Apr 22

[36] Raoofi S, Pashazadeh Kan F, Rafiei S, Hoseinipalangi Z, Rezaei S, Ahmadi S, et al. Hemodialysis and peritoneal dialysis-health-related quality of life: Systematic review plus meta-analysis. BMJ Supportive & Palliative Care. 2023;**13**(4):365-373. DOI: 10.1136/bmjspcare-2021-003182. Epub 2021 Jul 22

[37] Theofilou P. Quality of life in patients undergoing hemodialysis or peritoneal dialysis treatment. Journal of Clinical Medical Research. 2011;**3**:132-138. DOI: 10.402/jocmr552w

[38] Pai AB, Boyd A, Chavez A, et al. Health-related quality of life is maintained in hemodialysis patients receiving pharmaceutical care: A 2-year randomized, controlled study. Hemodialysis International. 2009;**13**:72-79. DOI: 10.1111/j.1542-4758.2009.00328.x

[39] Chuasuwan A, Pooripussarakul S, Thakkinstian A, Ingsathit A, Pattanaprateep O. Comparisons of quality of life between patients underwent peritoneal dialysis and hemodialysis: A systematic review and meta-analysis. Health and Quality of Life Outcomes. 2020;**18**(1):191. DOI: 10.1186/s12955-020-01449-2

[40] Kalender B, Ozdemir AC, Dervisoglu E, Ozdemir O. Quality of life in chronic kidney disease: Effects of treatment modality, depression, malnutrition and inflammation. International Journal of Clinical Practice. 2007;**61**(4):569-576. DOI: 10.1111/j.1742-1241.2006.01251.x. Epub 2007 Jan 29

[41] Merkus MP, Jager KJ, Dekker FW, De Haan RJ, Boeschoten EW, Krediet RT. Quality of life over time in dialysis: The Netherlands cooperative study on the adequacy of dialysis. NECOSAD study group. Kidney International. 1999;**56**(2):720-728. DOI: 10.1046/j.1523-1755.1999.00563.x

[42] Makkar V, Kumar M, Mahajan R, Khaira NS. Comparison of outcomes and quality of life between hemodialysis and peritoneal dialysis patients in Indian ESRD population. Journal of Clinical and Diagnostic Research. 2015;**9**(3):OC28-OC31. DOI: 10.7860/JCDR/2015/11472.5709. Epub 2015 Mar 1

[43] Diaz-Buxo JA, Lowrie EG, Lew NL, Zhang H, Lazarus JM. Quality-of-life evaluation using short form 36: Comparison in hemodialysis and peritoneal dialysis patients. American Journal of Kidney Diseases. 2000;**35**(2):293-300. DOI: 10.1016/s0272-6386(00)70339-8

[44] Ginieri-Coccossis M, Theofilou P, Synodinou C, Tomaras V, Soldatos C. Quality of life, mental health and health beliefs in haemodialysis and peritoneal dialysis patients: Investigating differences in early and later years of current treatment. BMC Nephrology. 2008;**9**:14. DOI: 10.1186/1471-2369-9-14

[45] Goncalves FA, Dalosso IF, Borba JM, Bucaneve J, Valerio NM, Okamoto CT, et al. Quality of life in chronic renale patients on hemodilaysis or peritoneal dialysis: A comparative study in a referral service of Curtiba–PR. Jornal Brasileiro de Nefrologia. 2015;**37**:467-474. DOI: 10.5935/0101-2800.20150074

[46] Kim JY, Kim B, Park KS, Choi JY, Seo JJ, Park SH, et al. Health-related quality of life with KDQOL-36 and its association with self-efficacy and treatment satisfaction in Korean dialysis patients. Quality of Life Research. 2013;**22**:753-759. DOI: 10.1007/s11136-012-0203-x. Epub 2012 May 26

[47] Al Wakeel J, Al Harbi A, Bayoumi M, Al-Suwaida K, Al Ghonaim M, Mishkiry A. Quality of life in hemodialysis and peritoneal dialysis patients in Saudi Arabia. Annals of Saudi Medicine. 2012;**32**(6):570-574. DOI: 10.5144/0256-4947.2012.570

[48] de Abreu MM, Walker DR, Sesso RC, Ferraz MB. Health-related quality of life of patients recieving hemodialysis and peritoneal dialysis in São Paulo, Brazil: A longitudinal study. Value in Health. 2011;**14**(5 Suppl. 1):S119-S121. DOI: 10.1016/j.jval.2011.05.016

[49] Moreno F, López Gomez JM, Sanz-Guajardo D, et al. Quality of life in dialysis patients. A Spanish multicentre study. Spanish cooperative renal patients quality of life study group. Nephrology, Dialysis, Transplantation. 1996;**11**(Suppl. 2):125-129. DOI: 10.1093/ndt/11.supp2.125

[50] Cook WL, Jassal SV. Functional dependencies among the elderly on hemodialysis. Kidney International. 2008;**73**:1289-1295. DOI: 10.1038/ki.2008.62

[51] Timmiers L, Thong M, Dekker FW, et al. Illness perceptions in dialysis patients and their association with quality of life. Psychology & Health. 2008;**23**:679-690. DOI: 10.1080/14768320701246535

[52] Zazzeroni L, Pasquinelli G, Nanni E, Cremonini V, Rubbi I. Comparison of quality of life in patients undergoing hemodialysis and peritoneal dialysis: A systematic review and meta-analysis. Kidney & Blood Pressure Research. 2017;**42**(4):717-727. DOI: 10.1159/000484115. Epub 2017 Oct 19

[53] Badri Man Shrestha. Peritoneal dialysis of haemodialysis for kidney failure? Journal of Nepal Medical Association. 2018;**56**(210):556-557

[54] Chanouzas D, Ping Ng K, Fallouh B, Baharani J. What influences patient choice of treatment modality at the pre-dialysis stage? Nephrology Dialysis Tranplantation. 2021;**27**(4):1542-1547. DOI: 10.1093/ndt/gfr452

[55] Chan CT, Blankestijn PJ, Dember LM, Gallieni M, Harris DCH, Lok CE, et al. Conference participants. Dialysis initiation, modality choice, access, and prescription: Conclusions from a kidney disease: Improving global outcomes (KDIGO) controversies conference. Kidney International. 2019;**96**(1):37-47

[56] Ho YF, Hsu P-T, Yang K-L. Peritoneal dialysis after shared decision making: The disparity between reality and patient expectations. BMC Nursing. 2022;**21**:268. DOI: 10.1186/s12912-022-01043-s

[57] Shi Y, Xiong J, Chen Y, Deng J, Peng H, Zhao J, et al. The effectiveness of multidisciplinary care models for patients with chronic kidney disease: A systematic review and met-analysis. International Urology and Nephrology. 2018;**50**(2):301-312

[58] Ino J, Kasama E, Kodama M, Sato K, Elzumi H, Kawashima Y, et al. Multidisciplinary team care delays the initiation of renal replacement therapy in diabetics: A five year prospective, single-center study. Internal Medicine. 2021;**601**(13):2017-2026

[59] Wang I-K, Yu T-M, Yen T-H, Yip H-T, Lai P-C, Li C-Y, et al. The impact of multidisciplinary pre-dialysis care on the outcomes of incident peritoneal dialysis patients. BMC Nephrology. 2022;(1):173. DOI: 10.1186/s12882-022-02800-z

[60] Spigolon DN, de Morales TP, Figueiredo AE, Modesto AP, Barretti P, Bastos MG, et al. Impact of pre-dialysis care on clinical outcomes in paeritoneal dialysis patients. American Journal of Nephrology. 2016;**43**(2):104-111. DOI: 10.1159/000444401

[61] Maffei S, Iadarola GM, Berta Scalzo L, Quarello F, Svoldi S, Vigilino G, et al. Indications from the first audit on peritoneal dialysis in Piedmont and Aosta Valley. Giornale Italiano di Nefrologia. 2011;**28**(2):188-194

[62] Blake PG, Edwina AB. Person centered peritoneal dialysis prescription and the role of shared decision-making. Peritoneal Dialysis International. 2020;**40**(3):302-309. DOI: 10.1177/0896860819893803

[63] Pommer W, Su X, Zhangh M, Liu F, Yin L. Implementing assisted peritoneal dialysis in renale care: A Chinese-German perspective. Kidney & Blood Pressure Research. 2018;**43**(5):1646-1654. DOI: 10.1159/000494679

[64] Povlsen J, Ivarsen P. Assisted peritoneal dialysis. Advances in Chronic Kidney Disease. 2007;**14**(3):279-283. DOI: 10.1053/j.ackd.2007.03.008

[65] van Eck van der Sluijs A, van Jaarsveld BC, Allen J, Altabas K, Béchade C, Bonenkamp AA, et al. Assisted peritoneal dialysis across Europe: Practice variation and factors associated with availability. Peritoneal

Dialysis International. 2021;**41**(6):533-541. DOI: 10.1177/08968608211049882. Epub 2021 Oct 21

[66] Giuliani A, Karopadi AN, Prieto-Velasco M, Milan Manani S, Crepaldi C, Ronco C. Worlwide experiences with assisted peritoneal dialysis. Peritoneal Dialysis International. 2017;**37**(5):503-508. DOI: 10.3747/pdi.2016.00214

[67] Walker CR, Tong A, Howard K, Palmer CS. Clinicians' experience with remote patient monitoring in peritoneal dialysis: A semi-structured interview study. Peritoneal Dialysis International. 2020;**40**(2):202-208. DOI: 10.1177/0896806081988763 8

[68] Broadhead WE, Kaplan BH, James SA, Wagner EH, Schoenbach VJ, Grimson R, et al. The epidemiologic evidence for a relationship between social support and health. American Journal of Epidemiology. 1983;**117**:521-537. DOI: 10.1093/oxfordjournals.aje.a113575

[69] BM Shrestha. Peritoneal dialysis or hemodialysis for kidney failure? Journal of Nepal Medical Association. 2018;**56**(210):556-557

[70] Joachim E, Gardezi AJ, Chan MR, Shin JI, Astor BC, Waheed S. Association of pre-transplant dialysis modality and post-transplant outcomed: A meta analysis. Peritoneal Dialysis International. 2017;**37**(3):259-265. DOI: 10.3747/pdi.2016.00011

[71] Korevaar JC, Feith GW, Dekker FW, van Manen JG, Boeschoten EW, Bossuyt PM, et al. Effect of starting with hemodialysis compared with peritoneal dilaysis treatment: A randomized controlled trial. Kidney International. 2003;**64**(6):2222-2228. DOI: 10.1046/j.1523-1755.2003.00321.x

Chapter 3

Innovative Strategies for Remote Patient Management in Peritoneal Dialysis: The Role of Artificial Intelligence

Ratnadeep Biswas

Abstract

The integration of artificial intelligence (AI) and telehealth in peritoneal dialysis (PD) marks a paradigm shift in chronic kidney disease care. In conventional PD practice, poor adherence to prescriptions leads to increased complications, hospitalizations, and mortality, while delays in care and inefficient oversight contribute to higher healthcare costs and workload burdens. Addressing these unmet needs is critical for improving patient outcomes. This chapter explores the evolution of remote patient management (RPM) in PD, emphasizing AI's transformative role in enhancing patient outcomes through real-time monitoring, predictive analytics, and personalized care plans. The historical progression from basic telemedicine to sophisticated AI-driven systems highlights the potential for reduced hospitalizations and improved treatment adherence. Despite the benefits, obstacles such as digital access, data security, disparities, and the need for specialized training persist. Ethical considerations, including patient autonomy and algorithmic bias, are also crucial in the responsible deployment of these technologies. As advancements in AI and telehealth continue, their role in managing PD is poised to expand, resulting in enhanced health outcomes and a better quality of life for patients.

Keywords: artificial intelligence, telehealth, peritoneal dialysis, remote patient management, chronic kidney disease, predictive analytics, personalized care, digital health, patient outcomes, healthcare innovation

1. Introduction

Healthcare is undergoing rapid transformation, with technological innovations significantly reshaping patient management, especially in the realm of chronic disease care. Among these, peritoneal dialysis (PD) represents a critical area where innovations in telehealth and artificial intelligence (AI) are creating new paradigms of care. As PD is predominantly home-based, effective remote patient management (RPM) has become essential for optimizing patient outcomes, enhancing adherence to treatment protocols, and reducing the burden on hospital systems. The incorporation of AI-driven technologies with telemedicine platforms is at the forefront of these developments, offering unprecedented opportunities to enhance the healthcare quality for patients undergoing PD.

In conventional PD practice, several unmet needs persist, hindering optimal patient outcomes. One of the most significant challenges is poor adherence to PD prescriptions, with studies reporting non-compliance rates ranging from 5% to as high as 50% in some cases [1–3]. This lack of adherence has serious consequences, including increased rates of technique failure, peritonitis, hospitalization, and mortality [1, 4]. Additionally, the delay in patient-provider interactions often results in insufficient anticipation and management of complications. Healthcare teams face challenges in adjusting prescriptions in a timely manner, leading to inadequate clinical oversight and reduced patient confidence. The excessive reactive workload placed on medical and nursing staff due to the lack of proactive monitoring also contributes to the inefficient use of healthcare resources and increased healthcare costs. These issues underscore the need for improved systems of remote patient management that can bridge these gaps and enhance the effectiveness of PD care.

The shift toward remote monitoring in PD is not merely a response to the challenges posed by the home-based nature of the treatment but also a proactive approach to leveraging technology for better patient outcomes. This is particularly significant in PD, where complications such as peritonitis, fluid overload, and catheter-related issues can arise suddenly and require prompt attention. AI algorithms, through predictive analytics, can identify patterns and potential issues before they manifest clinically, thereby improving patient safety and reducing hospitalization rates.

In Japan, for instance, the implementation of AI and IT in dialysis has revolutionized the approach to PD management. The development of systems like Sharesource, which enables remote monitoring and adjustment of PD settings, exemplifies the potential of these technologies to enhance patient care. Such systems allow healthcare providers to monitor critical parameters like fluid balance, blood pressure, and dialysis efficacy in real time and to adjust treatment regimens remotely, thereby reducing the need for frequent clinic visits and hospitalizations. Additionally, the COVID-19 pandemic has accelerated the use of telemedicine, underscoring its critical role in ensuring continuous care while reducing the infection risk for vulnerable patients [5, 6].

The potential of AI in PD management extends beyond mere monitoring. For example, AI can help in optimizing dialysis prescriptions by analyzing trends in patient data over time and predicting the best possible dialysis conditions tailored to individual needs. Tailoring treatment to individual needs leads to better health results and happier patients, as care is customized to their specific circumstances [5].

Although AI and telehealth have clear advantages for managing PD, there are obstacles to overcome, including data security concerns, limited access to technology, and the need for specialized training among healthcare providers. Data security, in particular, is a critical concern, as the sensitive nature of health data requires stringent measures to prevent breaches. Moreover, ensuring that both patients and healthcare providers are adequately trained to use these technologies is essential to maximize their efficacy and to avoid potential misuse [7].

As technology continues to advance, AI and telehealth are expected to become increasingly important in PD management, driven by the demand for efficient and patient-centered care. This chapter will explore the innovative strategies for remote patient management in PD, focusing on the transformative impact of AI and telehealth technologies. Through a comprehensive review of current practices, challenges, and future directions, it aims to equip healthcare practitioners with the insights and tools necessary to leverage these innovations for better patient care in the modern era.

2. The evolution of remote patient management in peritoneal dialysis

2.1 Historical perspective of remote management in healthcare

The concept of remote patient management (RPM) in healthcare dates back to the mid-twentieth century, when the first telemedicine practices began to take shape. Initially, these practices were rudimentary, involving simple communication methods like telephone calls to provide medical advice to patients in remote areas. The technology at that time was limited, and remote monitoring was practically nonexistent due to the lack of real-time data transmission capabilities [8].

In the 1960s and 1970s, NASA's STARPAHC project pioneered telemedicine by using telecommunications to provide healthcare services to the Papago Native American reservation in Arizona. This was one of the first examples of remote patient care and showed how telemedicine could expand healthcare access beyond traditional settings [8].

The rise of the Internet and communication technology in the 1980s and 1990s led to more advanced forms of telemedicine. During this period, healthcare providers began to explore the use of video conferencing and digital data transmission for patient consultations and remote diagnostics. However, the application of these technologies remained limited to certain specialties, such as radiology and psychiatry, where direct physical examination was less critical [9].

2.2 Development and adoption of remote patient management in peritoneal dialysis

The specific application of RPM in peritoneal dialysis (PD) began to take shape in the late twentieth century as PD emerged as a popular home-based therapy for patients with end-stage renal disease (ESRD). Initially, PD patients were required to keep manual logs of their treatment details, such as dialysate volumes, fluid output, and any complications encountered. These logs were reviewed during periodic clinic visits, which often left significant gaps in the monitoring and management of the therapy.

The first significant breakthrough in RPM for PD came with the development of early telemedicine systems that allowed for the electronic transmission of treatment data from the patient's home to the clinic. These systems, although basic, enabled healthcare providers to monitor treatment adherence and identify potential issues between clinic visits. However, they were still limited by the technology of the time, which often meant that data transmission was not in real-time and could be prone to errors [9].

The twenty-first century brought significant advancements in RPM for PD, largely driven by innovations in digital health and information technology. The introduction of automated peritoneal dialysis (APD) machines with embedded telemetry capabilities marked a major milestone. These machines could automatically record and transmit data on the dialysis process, including flow rates, ultrafiltration volumes, and dwell times. This automation reduced the burden on patients and improved the accuracy and reliability of data collected.

Furthermore, the integration of Internet-connected devices and mobile health applications allowed for real-time monitoring of patients. This development was particularly beneficial for identifying and managing complications early, thus preventing hospitalizations and improving overall patient outcomes. Companies like Baxter introduced systems like Sharesource, which allowed clinicians to remotely monitor and adjust PD therapy settings, greatly enhancing the effectiveness and safety of home-based dialysis.

2.3 Key drivers of remote management adoption

The adoption of RPM in PD has been driven by several key factors, including the need for improved patient outcomes, advancements in technology, and the increasing prevalence of chronic kidney disease (CKD).

Patient-centered care: One of the primary drivers of RPM adoption in PD has been the shift toward patient-centered care. Patients undergoing PD are often more vulnerable to complications and require constant monitoring to manage their condition effectively. RPM offers a way to provide oversight without the need for frequent clinic visits, thereby improving patient comfort and adherence to treatment protocols [10].

Technological advancements: The rapid growth of digital health technologies has been essential for the adoption of remote patient monitoring. Reliable Internet, widespread smartphone use, and smaller medical devices make it possible to accurately monitor patients from a distance. These technologies allow for the collection and analysis of large amounts of patient data, which can be used to customize treatment plans and improve health outcomes [11].

Healthcare cost reduction: Another significant driver is the need to reduce healthcare costs. Hospitalizations and in-person consultations are expensive, both for patients and healthcare systems. RPM can help reduce these costs by enabling early intervention and preventing complications that would otherwise require costly treatments. This is particularly important in the management of chronic diseases like CKD, where long-term care costs can be substantial [12].

Regulatory and policy support: The adoption of RPM has also been supported by changes in healthcare policies and regulations that encourage the use of telemedicine and remote monitoring technologies. In many countries, healthcare systems and insurance providers have begun to recognize the value of RPM in bettering outcomes and bringing down costs, leading to broader acceptance and integration of these technologies in routine care [13].

As the healthcare landscape continues to evolve, the adoption of RPM in PD is projected to grow, driven by ongoing technological innovations and the ever-growing emphasis on patient-centered care. The historical development of RPM in PD highlights the critical role of technology in enhancing the quality and accessibility of healthcare for patients with chronic conditions [8, 9].

3. AI-driven predictive analytics for early detection of complications in peritoneal dialysis

3.1 Introduction to AI and machine learning in healthcare

Artificial intelligence (AI) and machine learning are revolutionizing healthcare by allowing systems to analyze massive amounts of data and provide insights that were not possible before. In healthcare, AI-powered predictive analytics uses algorithms to identify patterns and predict future outcomes, allowing for early detection of diseases and complications. The integration of AI in healthcare is not just about enhancing diagnostics but also about improving patient outcomes through early interventions. AI models can analyze data from electronic health records, wearable devices, and even genetics to provide personalized healthcare solutions. Companies like Microsoft and Google are at the forefront of this transformation, developing AI systems that enhance the accuracy and efficiency of medical care [14, 15].

3.2 Predictive analytics in peritoneal dialysis

PD is a vital treatment for patients with end-stage kidney disease. However, complications like infections, catheter problems, and cardiovascular events can be serious. AI-driven predictive analytics can help by analyzing patient data to identify potential complications early on. For example, machine learning models can be trained on past patient data to predict the risk of peritonitis, a common and dangerous complication in PD [16]. By integrating data from various sources, including patient history, treatment regimens, and even lifestyle factors, these models can help clinicians intervene early, potentially reducing hospitalizations and improving patient outcomes [17].

Several real-world examples demonstrate the potential of AI for early detection in peritoneal dialysis. For instance, a case study showed how machine learning algorithms were used to predict early signs of cardiovascular events in PD patients. By analyzing data like blood pressure, heart rate, and medical history, the AI system could alert healthcare providers to potential risks, allowing for timely intervention [17, 18].

3.3 Benefits of early detection and intervention

By predicting complications, AI can help personalize treatment plans for individual patients, improving adherence and overall quality of life. This proactive approach not only enhances patient care but also reduces healthcare costs by minimizing the occurrence of severe complications [19, 20].

4. Automated systems for patient data collection and analysis

4.1 AI-powered tools for data collection

Artificial intelligence (AI) has transformed data collection in PD by introducing tools that automate and enhance the process. AI-powered platforms can gather and analyze large volumes of data from PD patients, reducing the risk of human error and enabling more sophisticated data processing. These platforms utilize algorithms to detect patterns in the data that may indicate potential complications, allowing for early intervention.

For instance, Baxter's Sharesource platform is an AI-driven tool that enables remote monitoring of PD patients [21]. It collects data from the dialysis machine and sends it to healthcare providers in real time. This data includes treatment adherence, fluid removal efficiency, and potential alarms indicating problems during the dialysis process. The AI system can analyze this data, providing insights that help healthcare providers make informed decisions about the patient's care plan [7].

Another example is the use of AI in predicting patient outcomes based on historical data. Machine learning algorithms can analyze past patient data to forecast potential risks, such as fluid overload. These predictive analytics are invaluable in tailoring treatment plans to individual patients, ensuring that each patient receives the most appropriate care based on their unique needs [22, 23].

4.2 Sharesource

Introduction to Sharesource platform: The Sharesource platform, developed by Baxter, is an advanced RPM system specifically designed for automated peritoneal dialysis (APD). It plays a crucial role in improving patient outcomes by allowing healthcare providers to remotely monitor and adjust treatment plans in real time, ensuring continuous and effective care. This system is particularly important for home-based dialysis patients, where regular clinic visits are less frequent, and early detection of complications is vital [24].

Two-way communication: A key feature of the Sharesource system is its two-way communication capability. After each PD session, the data is automatically transmitted from the patient's APD cycler to a centralized clinic system. This data includes critical treatment parameters such as fluid removal volumes, cycle times, and ultrafiltration efficiency. The information is relayed in real-time to the healthcare team, allowing physicians to assess patient progress remotely [25].

Remote prescription adjustments: One of the standout features of Sharesource is that physicians can remotely adjust prescriptions based on the transmitted data. If a patient's treatment needs to be modified due to signs of fluid overload, inadequate ultrafiltration, or other issues, the healthcare provider can make these changes instantly from their location without requiring the patient to visit the clinic. This significantly improves the flexibility and timeliness of care, ensuring that patients receive the correct dosage and treatment protocol at all times [26].

Flag system for alarms and alerts: The Sharesource platform employs a sophisticated flag system to alert healthcare providers about potential issues in real time. The system generates priority and high-priority alarms based on the data received after each PD session. These flags help nurses and physicians quickly identify and prioritize patients who may be at risk of complications. Some of the conditions detected by these flags include:

a. Poor patient adherence: If a patient fails to complete a prescribed dialysis session or skips treatments, the system flags this as a high-priority issue, prompting immediate action from the care team.

b. Catheter problems or poor drainage: The system can detect poor drainage volumes, indicating possible catheter malfunctions or blockages. This alert allows for a timely intervention, reducing the risk of infection or peritonitis.

c. Volume management concerns: Sharesource monitors fluid volumes during each dialysis session. If there is an issue with fluid retention or inadequate removal, it triggers an alert. This feature helps in managing issues like fluid overload, which can lead to hypertension or heart failure if left unchecked.

d. Treatment variables: The platform also tracks a range of treatment-specific variables, such as lost dwell time, lost therapy volume, early drain termination, and bypass of fill/dwell phases. These parameters are crucial in ensuring that the treatment is being administered properly and effectively. If any discrepancies occur, healthcare providers can intervene quickly to avoid long-term complications [27].

Data visualization (tables and graphs for clinical action): Once the data is transmitted, the Sharesource system provides detailed tables and graphs that visualize treatment data, making it easier for nurses and physicians to interpret the information quickly. This graphical representation of the data highlights trends and anomalies, allowing for immediate clinical actions. For instance:

a. Actionable insights: If a patient exhibits poor ultrafiltration over several sessions, the care team can visually track this trend and adjust the patient's prescription to avoid fluid retention or other complications.

b. Remote consultations: Based on the data visualization, clinicians may opt to schedule phone or video consultations with patients to discuss potential issues, offer advice, or recommend an immediate clinic visit if necessary.

This visual data helps care teams determine whether immediate action, such as calling the patient or requesting an in-person visit, is necessary to address any concerns raised by the flagged issues [25].

4.3 Integration of wearables and IoT devices in PD

The combination of wearable devices and the Internet of Things (IoT) has introduced a new way to monitor patients with peritoneal dialysis. Wearable devices, like smartwatches and biosensors, can continuously track vital signs and other health data, sending this information to healthcare providers through IoT networks. This real-time data collection is crucial for PD patients, who require constant monitoring to detect any deviations from normal health parameters that could indicate a complication [28, 29].

One innovative application is the use of IoT-enabled sensors that monitor the dialysis process itself. These sensors can track various aspects of the treatment, such as dialysate flow rates, catheter function, and the composition of dialysis fluids. This information is then transmitted to a central system where it can be analyzed in real-time, allowing healthcare providers to adjust treatment protocols promptly if any issues are detected [30].

A real-world example of this technology in action is a system designed to monitor potassium levels in PD patients. Potassium imbalances are a common issue in dialysis, and monitoring these levels is crucial for patient safety [31]. An IoT-based system can continuously measure potassium levels during dialysis, providing immediate alerts if levels fall outside of the safe range. This enables healthcare providers to intervene quickly, preventing potential complications such as cardiac arrhythmias [30].

4.4 Impact of real-time analysis on patient care

Real-time data analysis is a significant advancement in PD management, offering numerous benefits over traditional methods. With the ability to analyze data as it is collected, healthcare providers can respond to potential issues much faster than before, reducing the risk of serious complications and improving patient outcomes.

For example, real-time analysis of fluid balance data can help prevent both fluid overload and dehydration, which are critical concerns in PD. By continuously monitoring the amount of fluid removed during dialysis, healthcare providers can ensure that patients maintain an optimal fluid balance, reducing the risk of complications such as hypertension or edema [32, 33].

5. Enhancing patient adherence and reducing hospitalizations

5.1 AI-driven strategies to improve patient adherence

One of the significant challenges in managing PD is ensuring patient adherence to prescribed treatment regimens. Non-adherence can lead to serious complications, including infections, fluid overload, and ultimately, increased hospitalizations. AI-driven strategies are playing a crucial role in improving adherence by providing personalized, timely interventions that keep patients engaged in their care. For instance, AI algorithms can analyze patient behavior and send reminders for treatment sessions, medication intake, or lifestyle modifications tailored to individual needs. These reminders are often delivered through smartphones or wearable devices, ensuring that patients receive them promptly, even in their daily routines [34].

Moreover, AI systems can identify patterns of non-adherence and predict which patients are at risk of skipping treatments. By leveraging machine learning, these systems can adapt and offer more targeted support, such as educational content or telehealth consultations, which has been shown to enhance patient engagement and compliance [35]. The predictive power of AI is essential in addressing the behavioral aspects of chronic disease management, making it possible to intervene before non-adherence leads to adverse outcomes [36, 37].

5.2 Remote monitoring and its effect on hospitalizations

Remote monitoring in PD, powered by AI, has transformed patient care by providing continuous, real-time oversight of patient health outside traditional clinical settings. This shift has been particularly effective in reducing hospitalizations, as it allows for early detection and management of potential issues. For example, AI can analyze data from wearable devices and home dialysis equipment to detect early signs of peritonitis, fluid imbalance, or other complications. When anomalies are detected, healthcare providers can intervene promptly, often before the patient experiences symptoms severe enough to warrant a hospital visit.

Studies have shown that the integration of remote monitoring can lead to a significant reduction in hospitalization rates among PD patients [3, 38]. The constant flow of data enables healthcare providers to make timely adjustments to treatment plans, thus preventing the escalation of health issues that would typically result in hospitalization [39, 40].

5.3 Impact of remote patient monitoring on survival

A recent cluster-randomized clinical trial published in *Nephrology Dialysis Transplantation* demonstrated the significant impact of RPM on survival in patients undergoing automated peritoneal dialysis (APD). The study involved 21 hospitals, with patients divided into RPM-APD (403 patients) and conventional APD groups

(398 patients). RPM-APD patients, monitored using the Sharesource platform, experienced significantly better outcomes, with all-cause mortality notably lower in the RPM-APD group (33 deaths) compared to the conventional group (55 deaths). Additionally, cardiovascular mortality was reduced by nearly half, with 13 deaths in the RPM-APD group versus 24 in the conventional group [38].

The trial attributed these survival benefits to RPM's ability to provide real-time monitoring and early detection of complications such as cardiovascular issues and fluid overload. By transmitting data directly to healthcare providers, RPM allowed for timely interventions and prescription adjustments, preventing conditions from worsening. This proactive management not only reduced mortality but also lowered the incidence of adverse events and hospitalizations, showcasing RPM's potential to significantly enhance patient survival and overall clinical outcomes in APD [38].

5.4 Personalized care plans and patient empowerment

Personalized care plans, supported by AI, play a vital role in enhancing patient adherence and reducing hospitalizations in PD. By utilizing AI to analyze a patient's historical data, genetic information, lifestyle, and even psychosocial factors, healthcare providers can develop highly individualized care plans. These personalized plans are more likely to resonate with patients, as they consider the unique circumstances and preferences of each individual, making adherence easier and more sustainable [41, 42].

AI also facilitates continuous communication between patients and healthcare providers, offering support and adjustments to care plans as needed. This dynamic approach to care empowers patients by giving them more control over their treatment and making them active participants in their health management. When patients feel more involved and understand the direct impact of their actions on their health, they are more likely to adhere to their treatment plans [43].

Furthermore, personalized care plans reduce the likelihood of complications that could lead to hospitalizations. For example, AI can help fine-tune fluid management protocols for each patient, ensuring that they maintain the correct fluid balance and avoid the complications associated with both under- and over-hydration.

6. Cost-effectiveness of remote patient monitoring

RPM offers significant cost-saving mechanisms by improving patient outcomes and reducing the financial burden of complications and hospitalizations [3]. Below are the specific ways in which RPM reduces costs:

Reduction in hospitalizations and acute care needs: One of the primary drivers of cost reduction in PD is the early detection and intervention facilitated by RPM systems. Sharesource and similar platforms provide real-time data on patient adherence, fluid balance, and potential complications. By detecting issues such as inadequate ultrafiltration or catheter blockages early, RPM enables timely interventions, thus preventing serious complications like peritonitis or fluid overload that often lead to emergency hospitalizations. Makhija et al. estimated that in a simulated environment, RPM reduced the use of healthcare resources and avoided several hospitalizations, emergency room visits, and unplanned clinic visits, leading to total cost savings of approximately $23,364 in the U.S., $11,477 in Germany, and $7088 in Italy [3, 44, 45].

Optimization of prescription and treatment adjustments: RPM systems allow clinicians to remotely adjust PD prescriptions in real-time based on transmitted data, minimizing the need for frequent in-person consultations. This capability optimizes patient treatment, ensuring that issues like fluid retention or poor dialysis efficacy are corrected promptly, avoiding the escalation to more serious health concerns that require costly interventions. Ariza et al. showed that an RPM program could project cost savings of US$121,233 over 1 year in a cohort of 100 APD patients, driven by reduced hospitalizations, fewer peritonitis episodes, and a significant decrease in hospitalization days [46, 47].

Decrease in travel and clinic visit costs: Remote monitoring minimizes the need for regular in-person clinic visits, which reduces not only travel costs for patients but also the workload on healthcare providers. Patients who live in rural or underserved areas particularly benefit from RPM, as they can avoid the time and cost associated with traveling long distances to specialized centers. This reduction in clinic visits also frees up healthcare resources, allowing providers to manage more patients with the same level of staffing [48]. Uchiyama et al. demonstrated that RPM could reduce unplanned hospital visits, home visits, and emergency room visits significantly, leading to overall lower healthcare resource consumption [49].

Lower rates of technique failure: RPM systems provide real-time feedback on adherence and technique performance. Poor adherence is one of the major factors leading to technique failure in PD, which often results in the need to transition patients to more costly forms of dialysis, such as hemodialysis. RPM mitigates this risk by flagging non-adherence early and enabling providers to intervene before technique failure

Benefit	Description
Reduction in hospitalizations [38]	Early detection of complications reduces the need for emergency interventions and hospital stays.
Optimized prescription adjustments [46]	Remote data transmission allows for timely modifications to PD prescriptions, preventing serious health issues.
Decreased travel and clinic visits [48]	Minimizes the need for frequent in-person consultations, reducing travel costs and healthcare resource utilization.
Lower rates of technique failure [50]	Continuous monitoring and early intervention improve adherence and reduce technique failure rates.
Efficient utilization of resources [51]	Allows for the management of more patients with the same healthcare staff, optimizing resource use.
Improved adherence [39, 40]	Real-time feedback and reminders enhance patient compliance with treatment regimens.
Enhanced patient monitoring [30]	Continuous monitoring provides detailed insights into patient health, facilitating better management.
Timely interventions [12]	Early detection of issues enables prompt adjustments and prevents escalation of complications.
Cost-effectiveness [3]	Reduced hospitalizations and efficient resource use lower overall healthcare costs.
Better patient outcomes [38]	Proactive management and reduced complications lead to improved overall patient well-being and satisfaction.

Table 1.
Benefits of remote patient monitoring in peritoneal dialysis.

occurs. This not only improves patient outcomes but also reduces the long-term costs of managing technique-related complications [50].

Efficient utilization of healthcare resources: By allowing continuous monitoring of a large patient cohort without increasing clinical staff, RPM helps healthcare facilities operate more efficiently. Clinicians can monitor multiple patients simultaneously, responding only when a problem is flagged by the system, thereby reducing the need for constant oversight and optimizing staff resources. This efficiency translates into lower operational costs for healthcare providers, as the RPM system reduces unnecessary clinic appointments and ensures timely care for high-risk patients only [51].

Through these mechanisms, RPM proves to be a cost-effective solution in managing PD patients by reducing hospitalizations, enabling early interventions, optimizing treatment plans, and decreasing the overall healthcare burden. These cost-saving aspects make RPM a valuable tool for both patients and healthcare systems.

Table 1 summarizes the benefits of RPM in patients undergoing PD.

7. Challenges in remote patient management and AI integration

7.1 Data security and privacy concerns

RPM involves the transmission of sensitive health data, making data security and privacy a top priority. The integration of AI adds to these concerns, as AI systems require large amounts of data to work effectively. Ensuring the confidentiality and integrity of patient data is a major challenge. Data breaches, unauthorized access, and hacking are common risks that must be addressed. Strong encryption protocols, secure data storage solutions, and strict access controls are essential to protect patient information. Additionally, compliance with regulations like HIPAA is crucial to safeguard patient data and maintain trust in digital health solutions [52, 53].

Baxter's Sharesource platform has taken these concerns into consideration and it incorporates stringent data security protocols to protect sensitive patient information. All data transmitted through the Sharesource system is encrypted and anonymized to ensure that personal identifiers are permanently removed, safeguarding patient confidentiality. This level of encryption ensures that the data cannot be retrieved or accessed by unauthorized individuals, making the data transfer process fully secure and compliant with healthcare privacy standards such as HIPAA and GDPR [54].

7.2 Technology accessibility and the digital divide

The adoption of RPM and AI technologies is also hindered by disparities in access to technology, commonly referred to as the digital divide. Patients in rural areas or those with lower socioeconomic status may lack access to the necessary devices, reliable Internet connections, or the digital literacy required to use these technologies effectively [55]. This disparity creates a significant barrier to equitable healthcare access and can exacerbate existing health inequalities. Addressing this challenge requires not only improving infrastructure but also providing education and support to patients and healthcare providers to bridge the gap in technology usage [52].

7.3 Need for specialized training for healthcare professionals

The successful integration of AI in RPM depends heavily on the expertise of healthcare professionals. However, many healthcare providers lack the specialized training required to operate AI-driven tools and interpret their outputs effectively. This knowledge gap can lead to misinterpretation of data, inappropriate interventions, or reliance on AI without a full understanding of its limitations [56]. Continuous education and training programs tailored to the needs of healthcare professionals are essential to equip them with the skills necessary to utilize AI technologies effectively. Such programs should focus on both the technical aspects of AI tools and the ethical implications of their use [57].

7.4 Ethical considerations in AI deployment

The deployment of AI in healthcare raises several ethical concerns. One key issue is the potential for AI systems to undermine patient autonomy by making decisions that the patient may not fully understand or agree with [58]. Ensuring transparency in AI algorithms and maintaining a human-centric approach to care is vital to preserve patient autonomy. Additionally, there is the risk of bias in AI systems, which can arise from biased training data, leading to unequal treatment of patients. Ethical AI development must include diverse datasets and ongoing evaluation to mitigate bias and ensure fairness in patient care [59].

In practice, when Sharesource detects complications or inadequate dialysis, the treating team (doctors and nurses) invites the patient to the clinic. There, the patient is shown the AI dashboard, which visually explains the issue detected—such as poor ultrafiltration or catheter problems. The healthcare team collaborates with the patient, explaining the data and discussing solutions. This ensures transparency and fosters shared decision-making, helping patients understand their treatment and maintain autonomy in their care [60].

These challenges highlight the complexity of integrating AI into remote patient management and how current AI systems like Sharesource are tackling them. Overcoming these obstacles will require collaboration across multiple sectors, including healthcare providers, technology developers, and policymakers, to ensure that AI and RPM can fulfill their potential to enhance patient care while safeguarding against risks.

8. Future directions and innovations in PD remote management

As we look toward the future of remote patient management in PD, several emerging technologies and innovations hold the potential to significantly transform care delivery and patient outcomes.

AI advancements on the horizon: AI is continuously evolving; however, it is important to clarify that many current RPM systems, such as Sharesource, already have advanced capabilities. These systems can detect catheter issues, patient noncompliance, and other mechanical problems in real time. Therefore, rather than framing these features as part of a futuristic vision, it should be noted that current RPM technologies are already addressing these challenges effectively.

However, future AI advancements will likely enhance these capabilities by refining predictive models and integrating more complex data sets to improve early detection and preventive interventions. This could involve more precise predictions of complications like infection risks or long-term treatment outcomes beyond the mechanical or compliance issues already monitored today [61].

Vision for the future of PD care: The vision for future PD care is one where remote management systems are fully integrated into the everyday lives of patients, reducing the need for hospital visits and improving the overall quality of life. Wearable devices and even implantable sensors may become the norm, offering continuous health monitoring without disrupting the patient's routine. The ultimate goal is to create a fully autonomous management system where AI and machine learning not only detect but also prevent complications, making PD as safe and convenient as possible for patients [62, 63].

The future of PD remote management will likely see an ecosystem where technology, data science, and patient care are more interconnected than ever, paving the way for innovations that could dramatically enhance patient outcomes and transform the landscape of dialysis care.

9. Conclusion

The integration of AI and telehealth in the management of PD represents a significant advancement in the healthcare landscape, particularly for patients with chronic kidney disease. This chapter has explored the evolution of remote patient management RPM in PD, emphasizing the transformative role that AI-driven technologies play in enhancing patient outcomes, reducing hospitalizations, and improving adherence to treatment protocols.

The historical development of RPM in PD highlights the steady progress from rudimentary telemedicine practices to the sophisticated, AI-powered systems of today. These advancements have not only enabled continuous and real-time monitoring of PD patients but have also allowed for personalized care plans that cater to individual patient needs. By leveraging AI for predictive analytics, healthcare providers can detect complications early and intervene promptly, thereby mitigating risks and improving overall patient safety.

Although AI and telehealth offer benefits for managing PD, there are obstacles to overcome, including limited access to technology and the need for specialized training among healthcare providers. Ethical considerations such as mitigating algorithmic bias, are also critical in ensuring that these technologies are deployed responsibly.

Looking forward, the continued evolution of AI and telehealth in PD management promises to further revolutionize patient care. Emerging innovations, such as wearable devices and more advanced predictive models, will likely enhance the capability of RPM systems to provide even more accurate, timely, and personalized care. As these technologies continue to advance, they will become increasingly important in shaping the future of PD management, ultimately leading to better health outcomes and improved quality of life for patients.

Conflict of interest

The author declares no conflict of interest.

Thanks

Thank you for your time, and I hope this chapter has provided valuable insights into remote management innovations in peritoneal dialysis and the role being played by AI in its evolution.

Appendixes and nomenclature

PD	peritoneal dialysis
AI	artificial intelligence
RPM	remote patient monitoring
IT	information technology
ESRD	end-stage renal disease
IoT	Internet of Things
HIPAA	Health Insurance Portability and Accountability Act
GDPR	General Data Protection Regulation

Author details

Ratnadeep Biswas
All India Institute of Medical Sciences, Patna, India

*Address all correspondence to: ratnadeepbis2404@gmail.com

References

[1] Bernardini J, Nagy M, Piraino B. Pattern of noncompliance with dialysis exchanges in peritoneal dialysis patients. American Journal of Kidney Diseases. 2000;**35**:1104-1110. DOI: 10.1016/s0272-6386(00)70047-3

[2] Griva K, Lai AY, Lim HA, Yu Z, Foo MWY, Newman SP. Non-adherence in patients on peritoneal dialysis: A systematic review. PLoS ONE. 2014;**9**:e89001. DOI: 10.1371/journal.pone.0089001

[3] Sanabria M, Buitrago G, Lindholm B, Vesga J, Nilsson L-G, Yang D, et al. Remote patient monitoring program in automated peritoneal dialysis: Impact on hospitalizations. Peritoneal Dialysis International: Journal of the International Society for Peritoneal Dialysis. 2019;**39**:472-478. DOI: 10.3747/pdi.2018.00287

[4] Bernardini J, Piraino B. Compliance in CAPD and CCPD patients as measured by supply inventories during home visits. American Journal of Kidney Diseases. 1998;**31**:101-107. DOI: 10.1053/ajkd.1998.v31.pm9428459

[5] Nakamoto H, Aoyagi R, Kusano T, Kobayashi T, Ryuzaki M. Peritoneal dialysis care by using artificial intelligence (AI) and information technology (IT) in Japan and expectations for the future. Renal Replacement Therapy. 2023;**9**:31. DOI: 10.1186/s41100-023-00479-y

[6] Uchiyama K, Morimoto K, Washida N, Kusahana E, Nakayama T, Itoh T, et al. Effects of a remote patient monitoring system for patients on automated peritoneal dialysis: A randomized crossover controlled trial. International Urology and Nephrology. 2022;**54**:2673-2681. DOI: 10.1007/s11255-022-03178-5

[7] Virzì GM, Morisi N, Milan Manani S, Tantillo I, Gonzàlez Barajas JD, Villavicencio BD, et al. Scheduling of remote monitoring for peritoneal dialysis patients. Journal of Clinical Medicine. 2024;**13**:406. DOI: 10.3390/jcm13020406

[8] Agarwal S, Wilkie M. Remote Patient Management in Peritoneal Dialysis: Opportunities and Challenges. Basel, Switzerland: S. Karger AG; 2019. DOI: 10.1159/000496309

[9] Crepaldi C, Giuliani A, Milan Manani S, Marchionna N, Piasentin P, Ronco C. Remote Patient Management in Peritoneal Dialysis: Impact on Clinician's Practice and Behavior. Basel, Switzerland: S. Karger AG; 2019. DOI: 10.1159/000496317

[10] Thomas EE, Taylor ML, Banbury A, Snoswell CL, Haydon HM, Gallegos Rejas VM, et al. Factors influencing the effectiveness of remote patient monitoring interventions: A realist review. BMJ Open. 2021;**11**:e051844. DOI: 10.1136/bmjopen-2021-051844

[11] Boikanyo K, Zungeru AM, Sigweni B, Yahya A, Lebekwe C. Remote patient monitoring systems: Applications, architecture, and challenges. Scientific African. 2023;**20**:e01638. DOI: 10.1016/j.sciaf.2023.e01638

[12] Dworkin J. Remote Patient Monitoring. Tampa, FL, USA: Remote Care Partners; 2023. Available from: https://www.remotecarepartners.com/remote-patient-monitoring/ [Accessed: September 19, 2024]

[13] Serrano LP, Maita KC, Avila FR, Torres-Guzman RA, Garcia JP, Eldaly AS,

et al. Benefits and challenges of remote patient monitoring as perceived by health care practitioners: A systematic review. The Permanente Journal. n.d.;**27**:100-111. DOI: 10.7812/TPP/23.022

[14] Allam Z, Dey G, Jones DS. Artificial intelligence (AI) provided early detection of the coronavirus (COVID-19) in China and will influence future urban health policy internationally. AI. 2020;**1**:156-165. DOI: 10.3390/ai1020009

[15] AI-Driven Predictive Analytics in Healthcare Innovation. n.d. Available from: https://defouranalytics.com/ai-driven-predictive-analytics-healthcare-innovation/ [Accessed: August 24, 2024]

[16] Sapsitthikul T, Pongpirul K, Kanjanabuch T, Chuengsaman P, Punyabukkana P, Pratanwanich PN, et al. Optimizing home visits through machine learning for preventing peritoneal dialysis-associated peritonitis: A proof of concept study and results from PDOPPS. Clinical Kidney Journal. 2024;**17**:sfae136. DOI: 10.1093/ckj/sfae136

[17] Tanaka H. Machine learning-based predictive analytics for early disease diagnosis. Journal of Artificial Intelligence in Healthcare Medicine. 2023;**3**:20-28

[18] Prediction and Early Identification of Disease Through AI. n.d. Available from: https://www.siemens-healthineers.com/digital-health-solutions/artificial-intelligence-in-healthcare/ai-to-help-predict-disease [Accessed: August 24, 2024]

[19] Deepa R, Arunkumar S, Jayaraj V, Sivasamy A. Healthcare's new frontier: AI-driven early cancer detection for improved well-being. AIP Advances. 2023;**13**:115331. DOI: 10.1063/5.0177640

[20] Are Predictive Analytics Key to Reducing Costs, Improving Healthcare? One Expert Thinks So | Bryant News. n.d. Available from: https://news.bryant.edu/are-predictive-analytics-key-reducing-costs-improving-healthcare-one-expert-thinks-so [Accessed: August 24, 2024]

[21] Sharesource Remote Patient Management | Baxter. n.d. Available from: https://www.baxter.com/healthcare-professionals/kidney-care/sharesource-remote-patient-management [Accessed: August 28, 2024]

[22] Kumar Y, Koul A, Singla R, Ijaz MF. Artificial intelligence in disease diagnosis: A systematic literature review, synthesizing framework and future research agenda. Journal of Ambient Intelligence and Humanized Computing. 2023;**14**:8459-8486. DOI: 10.1007/s12652-021-03612-z

[23] Debnath S, Barnaby DP, Coppa K, Makhnevich A, Kim EJ, Chatterjee S, et al. Machine learning to assist clinical decision-making during the COVID-19 pandemic. Bioelectronic Medicine. 2020;**6**:14. DOI: 10.1186/s42234-020-00050-8

[24] Schmitt CP, Hothi DK. Remote patient monitoring in peritoneal dialysis. In: Warady BA, Alexander SR, Schaefer F, editors. Pediatric Dialysis. Cham: Springer International Publishing; 2021. pp. 315-321. DOI: 10.1007/978-3-030-66861-7_18

[25] Gebhardt AT, Mishra A. Two-Way Patient Monitoring in PD: Technical Description of Sharesource. Basel, Switzerland: S. Karger AG; 2019. DOI: 10.1159/000496314

[26] Sharesource. n.d. Available from: https://renalcareus.baxter.com/pd-hcp/sharesource [Accessed: September 18, 2024]

[27] Neri L, Di Liberato L, Alfano G, Allegrucci V, Appio N, Bussi C, et al. Precision medicine in peritoneal dialysis: An expert opinion on the application of the sharesource platform for the remote management of patients. Journal of Personalized Medicine. 2024;**14**:807. DOI: 10.3390/jpm14080807

[28] Verma D, Singh KR, Yadav AK, Nayak V, Singh J, Solanki PR, et al. Internet of things (IoT) in nano-integrated wearable biosensor devices for healthcare applications. Biosensors and Bioelectronics: X. 2022;**11**:100153. DOI: 10.1016/j.biosx.2022.100153

[29] Lu L, Zhang J, Xie Y, Gao F, Xu S, Wu X, et al. Wearable health devices in health care: Narrative systematic review. JMIR mHealth and uHealth. 2020;**8**:e18907. DOI: 10.2196/18907

[30] Dharini AL, Harshavarthini M, Hinduja M, Gokulalakshmi A. IoT based patient monitoring for peritoneal dialysis patients with DT approach. International Journal of Engineering Research & Technology. 2020;**9**:671-673. DOI: 10.17577/IJERTV9IS110265

[31] Choi HY, Ha SK. Potassium balances in maintenance hemodialysis. Electrolytes & Blood Pressure : E & BP. 2013;**11**:9-16. DOI: 10.5049/EBP.2013.11.1.9

[32] Alexandrou M-E, Balafa O, Sarafidis P. Assessment of hydration status in peritoneal dialysis patients: Validity, prognostic value, strengths, and limitations of available techniques. American Journal of Nephrology. 2020;**51**:589-612. DOI: 10.1159/000509115

[33] Fluid Overload in a Dialysis Patient | National Kidney Foundation. n.d. Available from: https://www.kidney.org/kidney-topics/fluid-overload-dialysis-patient [Accessed: August 28, 2024]

[34] Saber AF, Ahmed SK, Hussein S, Qurbani K. Artificial intelligence-assisted nursing interventions in psychiatry for oral cancer patients: A concise narrative review. Oral Oncology Reports. 2024;**10**:100343. DOI: 10.1016/j.oor.2024.100343

[35] Haleem A, Javaid M, Singh RP, Suman R. Telemedicine for healthcare: Capabilities, features, barriers, and applications. Sensors International. 2021;**2**:100117. DOI: 10.1016/j.sintl.2021.100117

[36] Gala D, Behl H, Shah M, Makaryus AN. The role of artificial intelligence in improving patient outcomes and future of healthcare delivery in cardiology: A narrative review of the literature. Healthcare. 2024;**12**:481. DOI: 10.3390/healthcare12040481

[37] Yang J, Wan J, Feng L, Hou S, Yv K, Xu L, et al. Machine learning algorithms for the prediction of adverse prognosis in patients undergoing peritoneal dialysis. BMC Medical Informatics and Decision Making. 2024;**24**:8. DOI: 10.1186/s12911-023-02412-z

[38] Paniagua R, Ramos A, Ávila M, Ventura M-d-J, Nevarez-Sida A, Qureshi AR, et al. Remote monitoring of automated peritoneal dialysis reduces mortality, adverse events, and hospitalizations: A cluster randomized controlled trial. Nephrology, Dialysis, Transplantation. 2024. pp. 1-10. (Online ahead of print). DOI: 10.1093/ndt/gfae188

[39] Milan Manani S, Baretta M, Giuliani A, Virzì GM, Martino F, Crepaldi C, et al. Remote monitoring in peritoneal dialysis: Benefits on clinical outcomes and on quality of life. Journal

of Nephrology. 2020;**33**:1301-1308. DOI: 10.1007/s40620-020-00812-2

[40] Tan SY, Sumner J, Wang Y, Wenjun YA. A systematic review of the impacts of remote patient monitoring (RPM) interventions on safety, adherence, quality-of-life and cost-related outcomes. npj Digital Medicine. 2024;7:1-16. DOI: 10.1038/s41746-024-01182-w

[41] Johnson KB, Wei W, Weeraratne D, Frisse ME, Misulis K, Rhee K, et al. Precision medicine, AI, and the future of personalized health care. Clinical and Translational Science. 2021;**14**:86-93. DOI: 10.1111/cts.12884

[42] Alowais SA, Alghamdi SS, Alsuhebany N, Alqahtani T, Alshaya AI, Almohareb SN, et al. Revolutionizing healthcare: The role of artificial intelligence in clinical practice. BMC Medical Education. 2023;**23**:689. DOI: 10.1186/s12909-023-04698-z

[43] Krist AH, Tong ST, Aycock RA, Longo DR. Engaging patients in decision-making and behavior change to promote prevention. Studies in Health Technology and Informatics. 2017;**240**:284-302

[44] Wallace EL, Rosner MH, Alscher MD, Schmitt CP, Jain A, Tentori F, et al. Remote patient management for home dialysis patients. Kidney International Reports. 2017;**2**:1009-1017. DOI: 10.1016/j.ekir.2017.07.010

[45] Makhija D, Alscher MD, Becker S, D'Alonzo S, Mehrotra R, Wong L, et al. Remote monitoring of automated peritoneal dialysis patients: Assessing clinical and economic value. Telemedicine Journal and E-Health: The Official Journal of the American Telemedicine Association. 2018;**24**:315-323. DOI: 10.1089/tmj.2017.0046

[46] Talbot B, Farnbach S, Tong A, Chadban S, Sen S, Garvey V, et al. Patient and clinician perspectives on the use of remote patient monitoring in peritoneal dialysis. Canadian Journal of Kidney Health and Disease. 2022;**9**:20543581221084499. DOI: 10.1177/20543581221084499

[47] Ariza JG, Walton SM, Sanabria M, Bunch A, Vesga J, Rivera A. Evaluating a remote patient monitoring program for automated peritoneal dialysis. Peritoneal Dialysis International: Journal of the International Society for Peritoneal Dialysis. 2020;**40**:377-383. DOI: 10.1177/0896860819896880

[48] Snoswell CL, Taylor ML, Comans TA, Smith AC, Gray LC, Caffery LJ. Determining if telehealth can reduce health system costs: Scoping review. Journal of Medical Internet Research. 2020;**22**:e17298. DOI: 10.2196/17298

[49] Uchiyama K, Washida N, Yube N, Kasai T, Shinozuka K, Morimoto K, et al. The impact of a remote monitoring system of healthcare resource consumption in patients on automated peritoneal dialysis (APD): A simulation study. Clinical Nephrology. 2018;**90**:334-340. DOI: 10.5414/CN109471

[50] Centellas-Pérez FJ, Ortega-Cerrato A, Vera M, Devesa-Buch RJ, Muñoz-de-Bustillo E, Prats M, et al. Impact of remote monitoring on standardized outcomes in nephrology-peritoneal dialysis. Kidney International Reports. 2024;**9**:266-276. DOI: 10.1016/j.ekir.2023.10.034

[51] Ali KIE, Mohamed M, Hamer R. MO700: Outcomes of remote patient monitoring among peritoneal dialysis population in the Covid-19 ERA. Nephrology, Dialysis, Transplantation.

2022;**37**:gfac078.037. DOI: 10.1093/ndt/gfac078.037

[52] Houser SH, Flite CA, Foster SL. Solutions for challenges in telehealth privacy and security. Journal of AHIMA. n.d. Available from: https://journal.ahima.org/page/solutions-for-challenges-in-telehealth-privacy-and-security [Accessed: August 28, 2024]

[53] LLC AT. Addressing the Challenges of Remote Patient Monitoring: Security, Privacy, and Ethical Considerations. Accuhealth Technol LLC; 2023. Available from: https://www.accuhealth.tech/blog/addressing-the-challenges-of-remote-patient-monitoring-security-privacy-and-ethical-considerations [Accessed: August 28, 2024]

[54] Global Privacy Policy | Baxter. n.d. Available from: https://www.baxter.com/policies-positions/global-privacy-policy [Accessed: September 18, 2024]

[55] Singh RP, Hom GL, Abramoff MD, Campbell JP, Chiang MF. Current challenges and barriers to real-world artificial intelligence adoption for the healthcare system, provider, and the patient. Translational Vision Science & Technology. 2020;**9**:45. DOI: 10.1167/tvst.9.2.45

[56] Davenport T, Kalakota R. The potential for artificial intelligence in healthcare. Future Healthcare Journal. 2019;**6**:94-98. DOI: 10.7861/futurehosp.6-2-94

[57] Tsvetanov F, Integrating AI. Technologies into remote monitoring patient systems. Engineering Proceedings. 2024;**70**:54. DOI: 10.3390/engproc2024070054

[58] Quinn TP, Senadeera M, Jacobs S, Coghlan S, Le V. Trust and medical AI: The challenges we face and the expertise needed to overcome them. Journal of the American Medical Informatics Association. 2020;**28**:890-894. DOI: 10.1093/jamia/ocaa268

[59] Ueda D, Kakinuma T, Fujita S, Kamagata K, Fushimi Y, Ito R, et al. Fairness of artificial intelligence in healthcare: Review and recommendations. Japanese Journal of Radiology. 2024;**42**:3-15. DOI: 10.1007/s11604-023-01474-3

[60] Burlacu A, Iftene A, Jugrin D, Popa IV, Lupu PM, Vlad C, et al. Using artificial intelligence resources in dialysis and kidney transplant patients: A literature review. BioMed Research International. 2020;**2020**:9867872. DOI: 10.1155/2020/9867872

[61] Davenport TH, Bean R. Five key trends in AI and data science for 2024. MIT Sloan Management Review. 2024. Available from: https://sloanreview.mit.edu/article/five-key-trends-in-ai-and-data-science-for-2024/ [Accessed: August 28, 2024]

[62] Iqbal J, Cortés Jaimes DC, Makineni P, Subramani S, Hemaida S, Thugu TR, et al. Reimagining healthcare: Unleashing the power of artificial intelligence in medicine. Cureus. n.d.;**15**:e44658. DOI: 10.7759/cureus.44658

[63] Yelne S, Chaudhary M, Dod K, Sayyad A, Sharma R. Harnessing the power of AI: A comprehensive review of its impact and challenges in nursing science and healthcare. Cureus. n.d.;**15**:e49252. DOI: 10.7759/cureus.49252

Chapter 4

Green/Eco-Dialysis

Sam Henderson

Abstract

The environmental impact of dialysis, especially Haemodialysis (HD), has been of increasing concern in research. This chapter will contextualize the concept of green/eco-Peritoneal Dialysis (PD) within the wider tradition of green nephrology and green dialysis. It will then provide calculations for electricity consumption and costs for patients in a typical case and in Gulf Cooperation Council (GCC) countries. The costs experienced by patients/patient households are discussed in the context of shared decision-making, equity, and relative environmental impact. The incremental financial impacts on home electricity bills for adult and pediatric PD patients are between 0.71% and 1.35% in the GCC. To further contextualize the impact of choosing PD in a green sense, a comparison between HD and Home-HD alternatives found that incremental electricity and water costs are much higher.

Keywords: environmental impacts, green nephrology/dialysis, equity in shared decision-making, cost burdens of peritoneal dialysis, health economics, continuous peritoneal dialysis, automated peritoneal dialysis, number of cycles, Gulf cooperation council (GCC) countries

1. Introduction

The contribution of healthcare to total carbon emissions is expected to be between 3% and 10% across international comparisons [1–3]. There is a direct link between the climate impact of emissions that warm the planet and health outcomes [4, 5]. It is expected both input and output variables create emissions at each stage from production to consumption [6]. Focus over the recent decades, such as on the Global Warming Potential (GWP) for Greenhouse Gas (GHG) Emissions, the extension of these mathematically to Carbon Dioxide Equivalence (CO_2eq), and relating everything to a weighted CO_2 equivalent value, has become a greater focus for policymakers and those in the healthcare space [7, 8].

In the UK, the contribution of water, waste, and direct energy consumption accounts for over half of the delivery of care segmentation [3]. Looking within the acute sector alone finds most emissions in all categories [3]. Emissions are produced now and impact the strength of future emissions [9]. This has been identified in literature through investigations of dialysis centers [10] and through international standards, such as the Task Force on Climate Related Financial Disclosures (TCFD) and the International Sustainability Standard Bureau (ISSB) [11, 12]. Meanwhile, definitions also sit with governments and policymakers [13]. The use of such blanket measures like an equivalent weight of carbon is criticized; the translation of an expected emission into warming the environment does not correlate [14]. However, it can be useful to view all impacts on the same scale, allowing for direct comparisons [1].

Nephrology services are considerably intensive given the acute nature of end-stage kidney disease (ESKD), treatment for kidney diseases, and Haemodialysis (HD) [15]. Peritoneal Dialysis (PD), by contrast, is seen as a lighter option in terms of its environmental impacts and comparable costs. This is quite natural given the differences: Treatment at home versus in a hospital, lower staffing ratios, no building upkeep related to treatment, and using the patient's own and already existing resources [16]. In other analyses of dialysis and its environmental impact, we can see there are key performance indicators, one of which is the electricity consumption measured in kilowatt-hours (kWh) [17].

1.1 The climate debate and nephrology

There are new fields or subcategories of study that aim to outline the various impacts of nephrology treatment options and services provided on the environment [18]. These created disciplines and traditions will contextualize the impact on the environment in terms of efficient provision of care when treating kidney diseases and establish guidelines on how to improve environmental sustainability [19]. When nephrology is considered a resource-intensive activity [15], it is suggested that regulations be established to address that intensity [20].

However, there are other considerations around how the burden gets counted in terms of measuring the impact and whether the provider is responsible for the impacts generated by the supplier of goods or whether the supplier is responsible [21].

1.2 Green nephrology

Green Nephrology exists to contextualize environmental impacts by identifying and discussing ways in which the provision of nephrology services for the treatment of kidney disease can be more efficient [22]. It will help mitigate the processes of climate change and subsequently reduce the future burden from carbon emissions on kidney health [22]. There are multiple perspectives in the sense of what emissions are included; we can look at nephrology as a field of medicine wholly influential in its own ecosystem or as a department in one or many hospitals [10]. We may look at wider environmental concerns that increase the pace of climate change and how impactful these increases affect trends in Acute Kidney Injury (AKI) and the incidence of kidney disease [23]. This Green Nephrology is located beyond single treatment options and considers infrastructure, social factors (transport), a dialysis session itself if appropriate, and the overall relationship between direct emissions and knock-on consequences [24]. This field discusses impact in terms of carbon dioxide equivalent weight, which will be "emitted" through various stages of care supply and provision [22]. Key authors have been branching into policy considerations and other decision-making advocacy areas aimed at creating a full discipline of Green Nephrology [18]. The key recommendations from this field lead to practical alterations in practice and help reduce overall expected climate impacts [25]. Moreover, it seeks to reduce the large and increasing burden of disease, which nephrology is associated with, by reducing the stressors on the environment, thereby alleviating some of the forecasted outcomes [23].

1.3 Green or eco-dialysis

Within green nephrology is green dialysis—or rather, the impact of the individual session of dialysis, whether HD, PD or the full patient journey in each modality [26, 27]. The dialysis session is at the heart of care and adjusting adoption rates to accommodate effective changes will reduce the overall impacts on the environment.

Not reducing what matters in terms of true carbon emissions, though, can have adverse consequences [28]. In this review we will look at the session in terms of its active consumption of various units, such as electricity [17]. Efficiencies can still be obtained by doing logical actions, switching machines off when not in use, and attempting to reduce consumable use or waste where possible; these will be meaningful and have long-lasting impacts [29].

Here the literature has primarily been applied to Haemodialysis due to its expected heavier nature versus PD [10, 15, 20, 23, 27, 30–35], although there are studies that have been produced, that do focus on PD in terms of carbon footprint as well [25, 29, 36, 37]. The body of work is often hampered by a lack of data or the need for substitution of certain values [38]. In works that do consider PD utility consumption, there are often estimations for the electricity consumed per session [25] or no estimation [37], which can make it difficult to have a firm grasp on what will happen when choosing PD in terms of additional burdens that may not otherwise be generated. Lastly, when we do understand the burdens, we will need to be mindful of the burden that is transferred to patients [27].

2. Peritoneal dialysis in the modern era

Healthcare's continuing ability to support demands in the market will continue to pressurize governments to act [4, 5]. Environmental impacts further compound the pressures with warming targets and points of no return [28]. Moreover, when it comes to PD, the flexibility of home care and the reductions in resource utilization will be beneficial from a budget perspective [16]. Environmental impacts are also judged less in PD versus HD, where they can be jointly assessed [29, 37]. Therefore, it would also be logical that PD offers an option for healthcare professionals to provide adequate care AND help the environment, in so doing performing "Green Dialysis." Less impact is not no impact [25], and there is always going to be room for efficient delivery of care in any health system [3, 38].

2.1 Modern peritoneal dialysis (PD)

In Modern PD we see informed decision-making become part and parcel of the Shared Decision Making (SDM) process [39]. Having the tools and information enabling informed conversation is paramount [40]. Continuous Ambulatory Peritoneal Dialysis (CAPD) is a notable therapy option; it tends to be cheaper than Automated Peritoneal Dialysis (APD) owing to the lack of a cycler and the flexibility of being able to do exchanges at your own convenience at different points in the day [16]. Of the therapy options, CAPD is considered the lightest, as it does not consume electricity outside of normal daily use [25]. So even when considering the dialysate production cycle, the delivery of the medication, and the disposal of the waste created [29, 41], it has a lighter impact [25, 37]. APD does consume electricity through using the cycler machine. It is done, often overnight, from between 8 and 12 hours, an average of 10 [42], and delivers a prescription that can be further tailored remotely if the feature is enabled [43]. When patients perform dialysis at home, their personal resource consumption will increase. This may be a slight increase given the cost of the therapy in total (this analysis), but it is an area where incentives can be deployed to encourage the home option, particularly with recent acute shocks such as COVID-19 [44].

This positions PD well, however, one of the many impacts on people in the last five years has been the sharp increase in bills related to energy, world turmoil has pushed supply-side factors and prices have risen [45]. Energy markets have ridden the waves of these increases, and the costs are passed on to consumers [45]. Here, PD and other home dialysis options can have material consequences for patients.

APD, when performed overnight, will incrementally impact a patient's energy bills. CAPD can, depending on availability in the market, be expected to have certain quality of convenience options too [36, 46], in the form of portable warmers. These will take a small electricity cost [46], and given it is reasonable to expect some impact, CAPD electricity costs are included for the purpose of our review.

2.2 The data gap - The patient perspective

The lack of data for professionals wishing to quantify these impacts [38] is apparent here. The options to resolve this are to use the details provided in other publications [25, 37], clinical literature where appropriate [42, 47], or to quantify some reasonable assumptions [36, 48]. There is very little in the way of finding out the expected power consumption of the APD machine, as manufacturers do not routinely publish facts such as the expected power consumption of their devices during operation. In this respect, as with other analyses, the electricity costs are seen as negligible [24, 49]. However, the financial impact, like the costs to patients, is seen as a barrier to choosing home dialysis modalities and should be addressed with the patient through education and discussion [50].

Societal costing is a factor that exists in cost-effectiveness papers and budget impact models [51]. In such comparisons between HD and PD options, the utilities (water and power together) are referred to and quantified collectively [16, 51]. Healthcare professionals, meanwhile, will want to have the fullest discussion with patients [52].

3. Patient perspectives - Overview of the analysis

The cost is incremental, and there is imperfect information. When considering patients who want to be informed in terms of what treatment options are available to them, the expected pros and cons are needed as part of that discussion [39, 52]. Outside of the therapy choice they are best indicated for, reasons for which will be outlined better elsewhere [42, 47], material and lifestyle impacts are key factors that can open or block therapy take-on [50, 52]. Household budgets are increasingly under constraints [45]; additional spending on healthcare can make the difference in the affordability of treatment often crucial to survival or the lasting impact it will have on household finances [53].

3.1 Peritoneal dialysis

PD does not require the direct consumption of water, a considerable factor in HD [35], and is known to have flexibility in further reducing impact [25]. This section will separate out the expected electricity consumption in units (in this case we refer to the unit consumed, denoted as kilowatt-hours [kWh]). The related cost of each unit has been outlined in other studies and can be localized to a country or utility company [20, 23, 25, 27]. Broadly, cost as a measure may take a physical monetary value (in a currency) or an environmental impact value (in terms of kilograms of carbon dioxide equivalence [Kg CO2eq]).

Through the provision of APD and CAPD modalities, electricity consumption is likely to occur; the use of the cycler machine as part of APD will result in the direct consumption of electricity [25, 37], and if the patient uses the quality of convenience device to warm the dialysate, there is an electricity cost associated [37, 48]. The rule of thumb is there are between 8 and 12 hours of dialysis needed to affect good dose adequacy [42, 47]. Meanwhile, CAPD is characterized by the number of exchanges per day [42, 47, 54].

3.2 Methods description

The analysis will identify a series of average or typical estimations for APD and CAPD modalities on a per-session basis, then extrapolate the results into yearly, annualized results.

The assumptions are that treatment will be seven days a week for a full year of fifty-two weeks. Real-term values derived per session will be multiplied by seven days for a week, multiplied again by 4.33 for weeks per month (52 divided by 12), and multiplied from monthly values by twelve for annualization.

There is a variance between the available data. We will employ averages through the summation of each option and dividing them by the number of options. There will be a series of low, average, and high estimated impacts created from each typical session detailed in this section, while later we will work only from the typical or average and suggest the use of the range of data if applying to different contexts as needed. Offering sight of the variability will also allow for contingency and flexibility when understanding reimbursement of costs, as some countries choose to offer [27, 55].

When localizing the costs for a particular country, an understanding (from an average perspective) of household sizes and the economies of the household will be required [56]. This is so we can have a relative perception of whether costs will be impactful or not [56]. Moreover, we will use standard economic data as reported from the World Bank [57–60] to enable discussions of the impact in context.

3.3 Results of the patient perspective per session

We are fortunate there are some reference points we can use for an understanding of the current costs to expect per session of PD. We have a few options to offer suggestions on the overall consumption per hour of APD machines. McAllister et al. [25] performed an investigative procedure with one APD machine and recorded its total Watt-hour (Wh) expectations for a single session. The UK has been harder hit than most countries due to the cost-of-living crisis [45]; efforts from the Welsh-Kidney-Network (WKN) [48] led to offering a request system for reimbursement with a local energy provider [55] through a cost calculator.

These options yield the estimations we outline, noting that the overall average in **Table 1** concerns per hour as well but assumes 10 hours per session. If we use these values as the best available data, we assume that APD can take place over 8–12 hours in a typical case [42]; therefore, we may outline the relative values as in **Table 2**. Taking the Wh values of **Table 1** and multiplying per hour can provide the variations of the expected potential consumption of electricity.

We may also be able to deduce a reasonable range through which we can posit various cost analyses to rationalize the prospective patient energy bill burden. From **Table 2** we may view the low (minimum) and high (maximum) estimations as laid out in **Table 3**.

If we wanted to account for different patient populations, i.e., different age demographics, it is helpful to view the potential options for electricity consumption from a stated average or typical perspective. In a well-cited handbook, overnight APD was suggested to be 10 hours per session per week for adult patients [42, 47]. Fortuitously, a recent environmental impact assessment in children offers us a glimpse into a variation in the number of hours for pediatric patients in the form of 11.2 hours per session per week [37]. Combining these expectations as the typical case with the average hourly consumption outlined in previous tables using the reference values provides us with the outcomes as per **Table 4**.

	McAlister et al. APD [25]	WKN APD minimum estimate [48]	WKN - Reimbursement (APD) [48]	Overall average [Noted below]
Per PD Session Per Hour (in Watts)	62.9 (52.5–78.7)	100.0	250.0	137.7

Table 1.
Key references for APD cycler electricity consumption per hour per session.

Number of hours per PD session per day	McAlister et al. [25] (Wh)	WKN APD minimum estimate [48] (Wh)	WKN - Reimbursement form APD [48] (Wh)	Overall average [Mean values] (Wh)
12	754.8	1200	3000	1652
11	691.9	1100	2750	1514
10	629.0	1000	2500	1376
9	566.1	900	2250	1239
8	503.2	800	2000	1101

Table 2.
Estimated variations in Wh consumption per session at different numbers of hours per session per day.

Range of unit consumption	Low	High
Wh per session	503.2	3000.0
Wh per session (Avg.)	1101.1	1651.6

Table 3.
Low and high estimations for Wh consumption per results and per the overall average.

DOI: http://dx.doi.org/10.5772/intechopen.1009183

	Number of hours per PD session per day [37, 42, 47]	McAlister et al. [25]	WKN APD minimum estimate [48]	WKN - Reimbursement form APD [48]	Overall average
Adult patient APD	10.0	629.9	1000.0	2500.0	1376.6
Pediatric patient APD	11.2	705.5	1120.0	2800.0	1541.8

Table 4.
Textbook and literature examples for APD electricity consumption in Wh in adults and pediatrics in terms of the expected number of hours.

Varying the time on the cycler to account for differences in residual kidney function or other factors that affect the prescriptions or compliance [42], we may outline the potential consumption as follows per session or per hour, as in **Table 5**.

There may be some start-up times for the APD machine that are considered within the values presented. This is because we are dealing with averages that also account for lower and upper limits, which already include the startup of the machine (expected for ~1 minute to reach operational functionality) and assume setup times are part of treatment time. Viewing this from a conservative standpoint, half an hour of setup time is accounted for within the overall session time and was assumed inclusive for reimbursement purposes [48]. Though for reimbursement purposes, the electricity consumption was higher than from the investigated values [25, 37, 48].

Lastly, for CAPD, it is expected that the treatment administration is done within resources with only the additional electricity coming from a dialysate warming device [36, 48, 55]; it is suggested [48] that it be more eco-friendly to have it always on. Therefore, we outline the expected consumption as **Table 6**.

The key values taken forward for the practical application are the averages in **Table 5** and the values in **Table 6** in Wh. We noted earlier we need kWh, which is 1000 Wh; therefore, the values in Wh will be divided by 1000 to be represented as kWh. No other changes are made to the resulting values.

	Per session			Per hour		
Range of unit consumption	**Low**	**Average**	**High**	**Low**	**Average**	**High**
Adult patient Wh	629.9	1376.6	2500.0	63.0	137.7	250.0
Pediatric patient Wh	705.5	1541.8	2800.0	63.0	137.7	250.0

Table 5.
Expected low, average (mean), and high estimations per session and per hour, Wh consumption for adults and pediatrics.

CAPD fixed power use assumption	Per hour	Per 24 hours per day
CAPD machine for warming dialysis fluid (Wh)	30.0	720.0

Table 6.
CAPD electricity estimation from treatment.

4. Gulf Cooperation Council (GCC) countries

We know conclusions from these derived values can vary considerably in this space [1–5, 10, 15, 20, 23, 27, 31–34, 36–38]. The analysis of electricity costs borne by the patient must be localized within a given jurisdiction.

In the previous section we covered the estimations; in this section we will cover the nuances of the countries and their related tariffs. Countries that make up the GCC states are Saudi Arabia, United Arab Emirates (UAE), Kuwait, Oman, and Qatar. Each of these countries is part of the Middle East region, which not only has higher than most daily temperatures [61] but also has a higher incidence and prevalence of ESKD [62]. A burden that is not only already impactful from a budgetary perspective but also is expected to rapidly and problematically increase over time [63].

Environmental sustainability has become an ambition for this region [64], and research on this region has quantified various societal or health impacts on the utilization of utility resources, namely electricity [65–71]. Moreover, factoring in the increasing prominence of issues around water scarcity, security, and usage [72–81], in addition to the often-referenced Water-Energy-Food Nexus [82–84], the GCC region offers a unique intersection across many disciplines.

4.1 Climate advocacy and participation in global initiatives in the GCC

Government-led climate initiatives in GCC countries will eventually exist to encourage participatory changes in the healthcare space given the high consumption of resources expected and within established national and international frameworks for transformation [85]. The recent hosting of the United Nations Conference to Combat Desertification (UNCCD) Conference of Parties (COP) 16 in Riyadh, Saudi Arabia, and the United Nations Framework Convention on Climate Change (UNFCCC) COP28 in the UAE are two example milestones reflecting regional participation in global initiatives [86, 87]. The growing importance of environmental concerns is going to continue to drive entities operating in these countries, whether public or private.

4.2 Healthcare systems in the GCC

Healthcare systems in the GCC, in addition, are undergoing national transformation projects in line with these ambitions [85]. Where outlined in recent literature, nationals in the GCC of their respective countries are fully covered for their healthcare costs, and have access to treatment in public, semi-public (privately owned state-contracted/budgeted), and private hospitals if they have additional health insurance or are participating in certain sectors of public life [88–100]. Expatriates are usually covered for healthcare needs through insurance schemes, and these are either mandatory or voluntary, while coverage of the specific treatment would vary according to the plan [88–100].

GCC countries have complex structures that inform their health services capacity, adoption rates for the modalities, the patient journeys, and how they differ from those in other markets [88–100]. Saudi Arabia has multiple health sectors and is moving toward accountable care organizations [101] to better manage the complexity. The UAE is structured for now with multiple organizations providing care for nationals [102], though signs point to consolidation at the federal level in the future. Qatar has a more symbiotic relationship between public and private provision of healthcare services, having semi-public entities cover 90% of healthcare [102]. Kuwait, Oman, and Bahrain have relatively straightforward health sectors, having one main payor through a main authority, which covers nationals within the urban centers and more rural areas [97–100]. Kuwait, though, it should be mentioned, has an additional mechanism (or desire if Afya is rescinded, or folded under the Ministry of Health Care as a pathway) for covering aged/retiree citizens under private care [103]. Comparisons worldwide are understandably difficult, reducing the ability to allow for more general frameworks to translate well across national (or sub-national) boundaries. The desire to pursue universal health coverage and increase access to care [88–100] means that for treatments like dialysis, the burden on budgets over time will increase.

4.3 ESKD patient journey in the GCC

The complex structures controlling the funding of care, which can be a substantial cost [62, 63], will have patient journeys in each case related to whether there are centers under direct public control or under a specific sector [104]. It was noted that between 94 and 100 percent of HD patients were living with family or friends during their treatment [104], a factor that seems logical to extend to PD. Most households are expected to have between 3 and 8+ people within the primary household [105], and as an assumption, we will assume an average household size of 4.4 people per typical household [56].

The split in modality choice for PD will also depend on the history and from where the patient is located geographically [104, 106–109]. From a recent study on the GCC PD populations [62], the percentage of patients with PD, the APD split, and the division between nationals and expatriates were reported. Multiplying the percentage stated and total number of PD patients, rounding up, gives the following populations (**Table 7**).

Kuwait, Qatar, and UAE have a greater than 50% split of PD patients who are expatriates [62] and 66%, 34%, and 87% APD patients respectively. Bahrain and Oman, by contrast, were entirely nationals, with higher APD splits (100% and 89%, respectively), and Saudi Arabian patients are mostly nationals as well [62], with between 3 and 4.5% expatriates covered and 79% APD adoption [62, 104]. Those expatriate patients would be using the private sector or charity to cover their treatment costs [104], so higher costs in general are less desirable, especially if treatment is not covered by insurance [63].

However, this analysis is a snapshot in time, only appropriate if elements used to localize the cost values remain reasonably true. If needed to apply to more specific circumstances, i.e., sessions within one clinic or other countries or sectors, the per hour or per session averages for kWh consumption from the previous section should be used and combined with whichever choices are appropriate to model cost and impact on the environment.

	Bahrain	Kuwait	Oman	Qatar	KSA	UAE
Number of APD patients	45	167	245	84	1014	134
Number of CAPD patients	0	86	30	161	319	19

Table 7.
Patient numbers for APD and CAPD derived from AlSahow et al. [104].

4.4 Electricity costs for GCC countries

Except for Kuwait, the GCC countries institute tier-based pricing tariffs (tier 1 charges on the first x kWh, tier 2 the next x kWh, and so on) through their related authorities for electricity, which will be calculated based on total monthly consumption in kWh [110–117]. Kuwait's electricity costs are a flat charge per kWh [115], so they remain the simplest of markets to address; however, there are subsidies in place for nationals to offset their electricity costs [61]. Bahrain incorporates subsidization for its citizens within their primary property but charges more for multiple properties [112]. Qatar outright exempts their citizens from paying the electricity bill for their primary residence [112], though as it was reported that ~76% of PD patients were expats [62] (thereby not exempt), we include their cost perspective. Saudi Arabia, for example, has a particular charging structure, which incorporates total amp load experienced by a customer's breaker as part of the monthly bill [110]. It is part of how the authority for electricity provision handles billing and services when directly interfacing with their customers [111]. UAE charges VAT at 5% on the total bill, while also applying a surcharge for electricity use in addition to the tiered tariff setup [116, 117].

4.5 Results

Figure 1 details the expected kWh consumption from a typical GCC household; the data is from 2014, where there was a reported Cumulative Average Growth Rate (CAGR) from 2000 to 2014 which can be extended to the values to assume for 2024 values. Taking total household consumption per month (kWh) from **Figure 1** as a base per household will determine the respective tariff used to calculate overall electricity costs (**Table 8**).

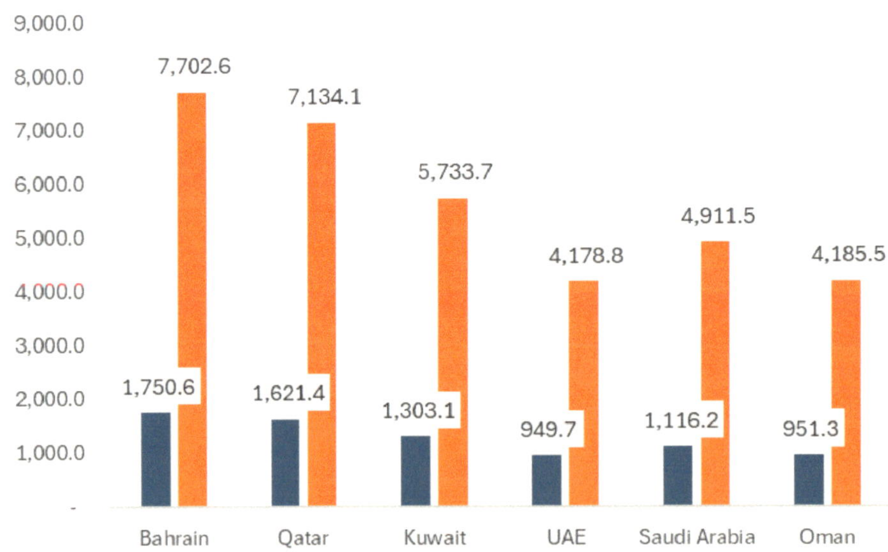

Figure 1.
Data from World Bank [58–60]- last reported kWh per capita for each country, adjusted to 2024 using reported 2000–2014 Cumulative Ave rage Growth Rate (CAGR) multiplied by the assumed number of people per household (4.4 MENA Average [53]), to get total Household kWh Consumption per month. Blue Bars—kWh Per Capita Consumption (per Month) World Bank [58–60]. Orange Bars—Total Household Consumption per Month (kWh).

Country	Respective electricity tariff per kWh (Local currency) [110–117]	Respective electricity tariff per kWh (USD)	Main unit local currency	Exchange rate local currency to USD [118]
Bahrain	0.016	$0.043	1 BHD	2.66
Qatar	0.180	$0.049	1 QAR	0.27
Kuwait	0.002	$0.006	1 KWD	3.24
UAE	0.320	$0.087	1 AED	0.27
Saudi Arabia	0.180	$0.048	1 SAR	0.27
Oman	0.018	$0.047	1 OMR	2.60

Table 8.
Respective GGC country electricity tariffs and relative currency conversion to United States Dollars ($, USD).

Using **Table 8** and the per-session unit consumption from **Table 5**, we can calculate the following average costs for APD patients (**Table 9**).

In this we outline the cycler's electricity consumption, assuming the time on cycler per session [37, 42, 47], and the consumption expectation derived from the literature [25, 48].

Repeating for CAPD. The costs for adult and pediatric patients on CAPD were the same regardless of demographic and the only variation was found in each country's respective tariffs, **Table 10** (below):

Extending the analysis to the total cohorts of patients reported in **Table 7**, we calculate the total average burden both in terms of kWh electricity consumption and in average cost for adult APD per country as follows (**Table 11**).

Adult CAPD patient cohorts are also considered and represent the following total average burden per country (**Table 12**).

4.6 Relative impact on electricity bills in GGC countries

To calculate the impact, we refer to available data in the public domain, finding the Gross National Income per capita per country from World Bank Sources [58–60]

	Adult patients		Pediatric patients	
Country	Per patient cost per month ($, USD)	Per patient cost per year ($, USD)	Per patient cost per month ($, USD)	Per patient cost per year ($, USD)
Bahrain	$1.78	$21.31	$1.99	$23.86
Qatar	$2.06	$24.76	$2.31	$27.73
Kuwait	$0.27	$3.25	$0.30	$3.64
UAE*	$4.53	$54.40	$5.08	$60.93
Saudi Arabia	$2.00	$24.03	$2.24	$26.92
Oman	$1.95	$23.41	$2.18	$26.22

Includes VAT and surcharge [116, 117].

Table 9.
Average patient consumption values on APD modality for adults and pediatrics versus expected consumption in kWh as per **Table 5**.

	Adult and pediatric patients	
Country	Per patient cost per month ($, USD)	Per patient cost per year ($, USD)
Bahrain	$0.93	$11.14
Qatar	$1.08	$12.95
Kuwait	$0.14	$1.70
UAE*	$2.37	$28.45
Saudi Arabia	$1.05	$12.57
Oman	$1.02	$12.24

Includes VAT and surcharge [116, 117].

Table 10.
Average patient consumption values on CAPD modality for adults and pediatrics versus expected consumption in kWh as per **Table 6**.

Country	Number of adult APD patients nationally	Total estimated average yearly electricity consumption on APD (kWh)	Total estimated average yearly electricity cost on APD ($, USD)
Bahrain	45	22,531.91	$958.80
Qatar	84	42,059.56	$2079.87
Kuwait	167	83,618.42	$542.17
UAE*	134	67,095.02	$7289.56
Saudi Arabia	1014	507,719.00	$24,370.51
Oman	245	122,673.72	$5735.49

Table 11.
Average electricity consumption (kWh) and electricity cost to patients for adult APD patient cohorts nationally.

Country	Number of adult CAPD patients nationally	Total estimated average yearly electricity consumption on CAPD (kWh)	Total estimated average yearly electricity cost on CAPD ($, USD)
Bahrain	—	N/A	N/A
Qatar	161	42,162.42	$2084.95
Kuwait	86	22,521.54	$146.03
UAE*	19	4975.69	$540.59
Saudi Arabia	319	83,539.21	$4009.88
Oman	30	7856.35	$367.32

Table 12.
Average electricity consumption (kWh) and electricity cost to patients for adult CAPD patient cohorts nationally.

and comparing them with the calculations in **Table 9**. We assume the patient loses no productivity from choosing PD and would have access to income in line with the average. The results are as follows (**Table 13**).

Deficiencies in productivity or loss of income will strain the financial aspects patients will be facing. It is likely that patients will already be experiencing these and other stressors because of their condition [50, 52]. The incremental impact on the

Country	Gross National Income (GNI) per capita	Total average cost of electricity per typical household	Total % of electricity costs versus GNI per household	Total average incremental cost of adult APD	Total average incremental cost of adult APD in % of total bill
Bahrain	$53,502	$2241.78	4.19%	$21.31	0.94%
Qatar	$108,491	$3442.22	3.17%	$24.76	0.71%
Kuwait	$56,132	$446.11	0.79%	$3.25	0.72%
UAE	$69,134	$4515.03	6.53%	$54.40	1.19%
Saudi Arabia	$52,372	$2896.21	5.53%	$24.03	0.83%
Oman	$34,272	$1849.57	5.40%	$23.41	1.25%

Table 13.
Comparisons of average electricity costs, average percentage impact of electricity costs, average adult APD incremental electricity cost, and average percentage impact on total electricity bills from APD.

electricity bills that could be expected for a patient choosing PD, on average, will be between 0.71% and 1.25% additional per year in costs. While **Table 12** reported for adult APD, it is likely between 0.81% and 1.35% for pediatric patients (due to the increased time on cycler [42, 47]). In CAPD, the average impact is likely to be between 0.38% and 0.70% for adults and pediatrics.

5. Shared decision making: The relative implications of PD, equity in dialysis and the environment

Shared Decision Making (SDM) is the practice of making sure the patient is having an informed conversation around the choice of therapy [39]. The mindset shift relates to applying as much empathy to the process as possible to affect the best outcomes so that the duty of care to inform fully is fulfilled [39, 40, 54]. The electricity consumption for CAPD is assumed to be nil and a boon for choosing the modality in SDM discussions, while not being seen as a negative in terms of SDM for APD [54]. The patient's financial stress must be a consideration [119], even if the costs are small.

5.1 Comparisons directly with the alternative HD options

The patient may be put off choosing PD if the incremental costs are discussed in isolation. Alternative dialysis treatment options such as In-Center Haemodialysis (ICHD) or Home Haemodialysis (HHD) should also be included in discussing dialysis choices. HD modalities have additional costs related to electricity and water consumption along with other significant out-of-pocket expenses if performed at home rather than in a clinic or center [120].

To cover this briefly, we note a recent study assessing the differences in HD modalities in Saudi Arabia [35] (adults undergoing ICHD and Hemodiafiltration (HDF) specifically) and report the following electricity and water consumption per patient per year (**Table 14**):

The use of a Reverse Osmosis (RO) machine, which would be used to facilitate the production of the high-quality dialysis water used during each session and be required for disinfection [27], was not included in the study as the comparisons were solely within HD, and the water production and electricity usage were considered part of the clinic's overheads regardless [35].

Extending this work, combining it with the available information we have considered in this review [48, 56], we see that electricity consumption is expected to drastically increase to 17.42 kWh per patient per week [48], and water consumption would be as high as 3.15 cubic meters (m^3) per patient per week [48]. HHD has such a large water cost due to the RO system and the process of rejecting up to 75% of water as non-viable and therefore increasing consumption drastically [24].

Annualizing the consumption and the cost, comparing to the household totals using this chapter's methods, yields the following results (**Table 15**):

With the per patient per week consumption of 17.42 kWh [48], the per year consumption is 905.14 kWh, and the cost would equate to $43.45 or 1.5% incremental expenditure on electricity bills. Saudi Arabia's household water consumption has been estimated to be 300 L/day [122]. When annualized, this means a household consumption of 491.04 m3 and $695.91. Calculating the water use, though, shows an incremental cost of $228.06 or 24.7%. Overall, a patient on HHD would be expected to incur, on average, $271.51 or 7.0% incremental expenditure on bills per year.

Figure 2 highlights the differences in percentage incremental cost impacts from HHD, HD, and PD modalities. Water and electricity are charged separately so the incremental costs are considered separate from each bill's perspective. ICHD patients are part of a clinic or ward's cohort, so there is some mitigation through economies of scale. In HHD, the patient will have significantly increased water bills, which will

Consumption unit	Adult patient yearly consumption, HD, on average [35]	Adult patient yearly cost, HD, on average HD (USD) [35]*
Electricity, kWh	461.00	$22.13
Water, m^3	29.24	$35.08
Total	N/A	$57.21

**Costs adjusted for residential tariffs derived from this chapter's reviewed sources [110, 111, 121].*

Table 14.
Average per patient yearly consumption in respective utility units for electricity and water in Saudi Arabia during a typical dialysis session within a clinic [35].

Country	Total average household cost (USD)	Adult HHD patient, on average, unit [35, 48]	Average adult HHD incremental cost (USD)	Total average incremental cost of HHD in % of total bill
Electricity (kWh, USD cost)	$2896.21	905.14	$43.45	1.5%
Water (m^3, USD cost)	$695.91	163.78	$228.06	24.7%
Total (USD cost)	$3592.12	N/A	$271.51	7.0%

Table 15.
Comparisons of average electricity and water costs for home haemodialysis in Saudi Arabia with average percentage impact on total electricity and water bills.

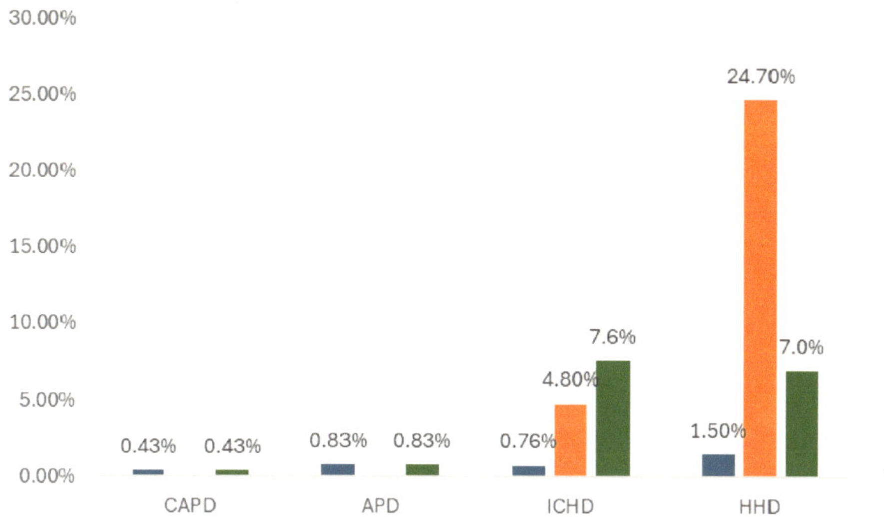

Figure 2.
Data from respective impacts in percentage terms of incremental spending on each bill and combined Water and Electricity in Total in Saudi Arabia. Blue Bars—Average Incremental Cost in % of total bill, Electricity. Orange Bars—Average Incremental Cost in % of total bill, Water. Green Bars—Average Incremental Cost in % of total bill, Total.

increase the overall utility bills commensurately. This should adequately confirm that PD costs are more manageable and re-center informed choice around the medical benefits of the available options.

5.2 Equity in dialysis treatment

There is bidirectionality of decision-making between patients and physicians [123], affording the patients themselves the chance to become aware of cost impacts during the Option Talk phase [39, 123]. Knowing that this decision rests in part with them [124] and expanding these discussions as appropriate should lead to better choice satisfaction [50, 52, 54, 125].

The impact of HHD has already raised questions around equity due to the shift in budget from payor/provider to household [27, 53]. In all cases, healthcare professionals will strive to provide the best care with the best outcomes [119, 126], but the incremental impact of the electricity consumption from a choice to utilize APD or CAPD was not enough to shift any of the typical scenarios into a higher tariff tier for any GCC country.

The same could not be said with HHD; the typical household water tariff increased in Saudi Arabia to the next tier due to the increase in water consumption, moving from between 31 and 45 m3 to between 46 and 60 m3 [121], the impact of which is a difference of $31.53 per year. Additionally, HHD requires home installation costs, including the physical home installation of the machines, additional staff costs, and inconsistent protocols across countries limiting remote care options [16, 27, 32, 52].

The overall cost of treatment is high [63]. Dialysis patients can receive a reimbursement to cover the costs of home care in terms of dialysis utility consumption as in Canada [27], Australia [10, 25, 31, 33], and per the reference example in Wales [48, 55]. Reimbursement can further unlock the pathway for patients to achieve the

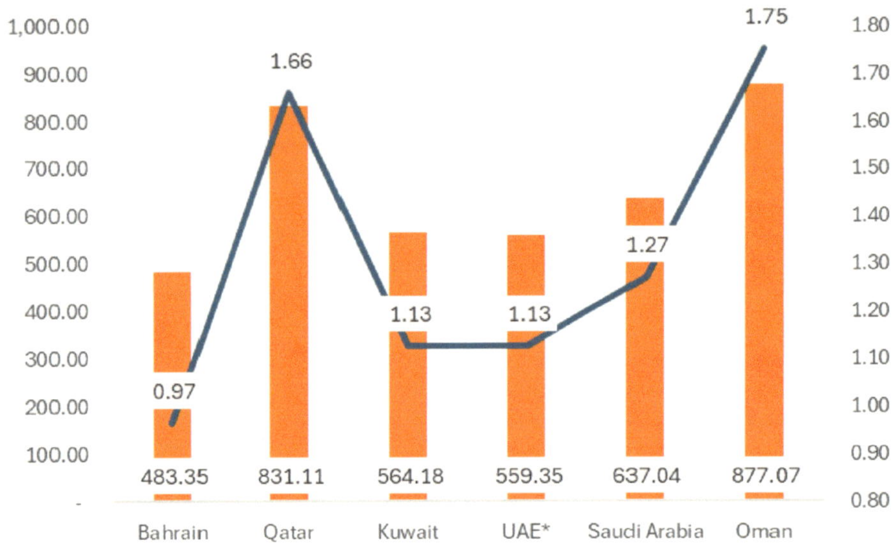

Figure 3.
Data from International Energy Association (IEA) derived kg per kWh from Emissions per electricity production and total electricity production [127–132]. Orange Bars—Total Estimated Average Yearly Electricity based Carbon. Emission per Patient (Kg CO_2). Blue Line—Kg CO_2 per kWh.

outcomes they will prefer and is likely to offset some of the equity challenges. Yet in comparison to HHD, PD remains cheaper to implement.

5.3 Social cost of carbon

Given values outlined in **Tables 11** and **12**, should the discussions around the intensity and impact on the environment from dialysis also be shifted to patients through tax (dis)incentives, then attention must also be paid to the relative carbon impact as is covered in the literature [10, 23, 25, 27, 36].

Using respective country data from the International Energy Agency (IEA) profiles online regarding emissions and electricity generation, we can assume an impact of kg carbon emissions per every kWh consumed (**Figure 3**) [127–132].

When compared to other markets where assessments of PD carbon footprints have been made, such as China [36] and Australia [25], the carbon emissions are broadly in line with one another (1.19 kg and 1.29 kg CO_2 per kWh, respectively [133, 134]). However, as we have also mentioned, this is not necessarily going to tackle climate change unless the measures that you are reducing have a direct impact on reducing carbon dioxide emissions [28].

It will be the case that reducing the prescription or time on cycler will have an impact on reducing the carbon footprint of PD [25], but this should always remain in the hands of the treating physicians to judge what is best for the patients in their care [25, 119].

Applying a cost to carbon consumption would also require caution, as reporting the carbon emissions in CO_2eq can be done with different perspectives on the way to the household. It therefore needs a comprehensive approach to judge the correct impact at the correct point in the lifecycle. Furthermore, the adoption of home-based dialysis has been shown to reduce the consumption of healthcare resources either in hospitals [43] or through telemedicine-based savings [43, 126]; attention is needed here too to avoid laboring the patient with costs otherwise accounted for.

6. Conclusion

The hope from this chapter is that there are clearer estimations of the cost and access to starting assumptions to improve decision-making. The objective was to understand what costs and burdens a typical patient may encounter so that there is greater information available for the needed SDM conversations with patients.

The wider implications of an increase in patients on therapy options will affect any given country. The imperative to gather the actual running cost during a session of dialysis should be clear, and further research is needed.

Since the prevalence of ESKD in the Middle East region will continue to rise and therefore contribute to climate change through increased volumes of sessions, further research will be necessary to monitor the overall environmental and societal burden PD and other dialysis represent.

The consideration of and preparation for the electricity-based costs can form a good base from which other conversations around the benefits of PD can occur with patients, across providers, in healthcare sectors, and with manufacturers or suppliers directly. The application of this research, which focuses on the specified unit consumption within a session, will be scalable. Comparable to other contexts and configurations in terms of costs, consumption, and economics.

Overall, given the low incremental impact on electricity bills identified, the impact of choosing PD remains a manageable and viable option in the provision of home-based dialysis care.

Conflict of interest

Sam Henderson is an employee of Baxter AG Scientific Office based in the United Arab Emirates, which sells and promotes dialysis equipment and consumables.

Author details

Sam Henderson
Scientific Office, Baxter AG, Dubai, United Arab Emirates

*Address all correspondence to: sam_hendersen@baxter.com

References

[1] Pichler PP et al. International comparison of health care carbon footprints. Environmental Research Letters. 2019;**14**(6):064004

[2] Blankestijn PJ et al. ERA-EDTA invests in transformation to greener health care. Nephrology Dialysis Transplantation. 2018;**33**(6):901-903

[3] Tennison I et al. Health care's response to climate change: A carbon footprint assessment of the NHS in England. The Lancet Planetary Health. 2021;**5**(2):e84-e92

[4] Romanello M et al. The 2023 report of the lancet countdown on health and climate change: The imperative for a health-centred response in a world facing irreversible harms. The Lancet. 2023;**402**(10419):2346-2394

[5] Romanello M et al. The 2024 report of the lancet countdown on health and climate change: Facing record-breaking threats from delayed action. The Lancet. 2024;**404**(10465):1847-1896

[6] Piccoli GB et al. Eco-dialysis: The financial and ecological costs of dialysis waste products: Is a 'cradle-to-cradle' model feasible for planet-friendly haemodialysis waste management? Nephrology Dialysis Transplantation. 2015;**30**(6):1018-1027

[7] Shine KP et al. Comparing the climate effect of emissions of short-and long-lived climate agents. Philosophical Transactions of the Royal Society A: Mathematical, Physical and Engineering Sciences. 1856;**2007**(365):1903-1914

[8] Campbell-Lendrum D et al. Climate change and health: Three grand challenges. Nature Medicine. 2023;**29**(7):1631-1638

[9] Collins WJ et al. Stable climate metrics for emissions of short and long-lived species—Combining steps and pulses. Environmental Research Letters. 2020;**15**(2):024018

[10] Barraclough KA et al. Updating the data: The resource consumption of modern-day hemodialysis systems. Kidney International Reports. 2024;**9**(5):1521-1524

[11] Task Force on Climate Related Financial Disclosures Status Report. Basel, Switzerland; October 2023. Available from: https://assets.bbhub.io/company/sites/60/2023/09/2023-Status-Report.pdf [Accessed: January 24, 2024]

[12] The IFRS Foundation, International Sustainability Standards Board Issued Standards. London, UK. 2023. Available from: https://www.ifrs.org/issued-standards/ifrs-sustainability-standards-navigator/sustainability-pdf-collection/?language=en&issue-type=%2Fcontent%2Fcq%3Atags%2Fifrs%2Fproduction%2Fissue-type%2Fissued&year=2023&layer=%2Fcontent%2Fcq%3Atags%2Fifrs%2Fproduction%2Fstandard-layer%2Fbase [Accessed: January 24, 2024]

[13] Hodnebrog Ø et al. Updated global warming potentials and radiative efficiencies of halocarbons and other weak atmospheric absorbers. Reviews of Geophysics. 2020;**58**(3):e2019RG000691

[14] Laurent A et al. Limitations of carbon footprint as indicator of environmental sustainability. Environmental Science & Technology. 2012;**46**(7):4100-4108

[15] Wieliczko M et al. Eco-dialysis: Fashion or necessity. International

Urology and Nephrology. 2020;**52**:519-523

[16] Roberts G et al. Current costs of dialysis modalities: A comprehensive analysis within the United Kingdom. Peritoneal Dialysis International. 2022;**42**(6):578-584

[17] Blankestijn PJ et al. Nephrology: Achieving sustainability. Nephrology Dialysis Transplantation. 2020;**35**(12):2030-2033

[18] Stigant CE et al. The necessity of environmentally sustainable kidney care. Canadian Journal of Kidney Health and Disease. 2023;**10**:20543581231166484

[19] Vanholder R et al. The European green deal and nephrology: A call for action by the European kidney health alliance. Nephrology Dialysis Transplantation. 2023;**38**(5):1080-1088

[20] Bendine G et al. Haemodialysis therapy and sustainable growth: A corporate experience in France. Nephrology Dialysis Transplantation. 2020;**35**(12):2154-2160

[21] Greenhouse Gas Protocol—Revised Corporate Standards. World Resources Institute; 2024. Available from: https://ghgprotocol.org/standards-guidance; [Accessed: December 16]

[22] De Chiara L et al. Green nephrology: An editor's journey. Journal of Nephrology. 2024;**37**(1):3-5

[23] Nagai K et al. Sustainability in dialysis therapy: Japanese local and global challenge. Renal Replacement Therapy. 2021;7:1-6

[24] Gauly A et al. Advanced hemodialysis equipment for more eco-friendly dialysis. International Urology and Nephrology. 2022;**54**(5):1059-1065

[25] McAlister S et al. The carbon footprint of peritoneal dialysis in Australia. Journal of the American Society of Nephrology. 2024;**10**:681

[26] Wandler S et al. Energy consumption models in dialysis clinics for agent-based decision support. International Journal of Simulation and Process Modelling. 2020;**15**(1-2):170-188

[27] Nickel M et al. Estimating patient-borne water and electricity costs in home hemodialysis: A simulation. Canadian Medical Association Open Access Journal. 2017;**5**(1):E61-E65

[28] Pierrehumbert RT. Short-lived climate pollution. Annual Review of Earth and Planetary Sciences. 2014;**42**(1):341-379

[29] Michalski R. Renal replacement therapy and environmental risks. Renal Disease and Transplantation Forum. 2024;**17**(1):19-24

[30] Yau A et al. Addressing the environmental impact of kidney care. American Journal of Kidney Diseases. 2021;**77**(3):406-409

[31] Barraclough KA et al. Green dialysis survey: Establishing a baseline for environmental sustainability across dialysis facilities in Victoria, Australia. Nephrology. 2019;**24**(1):88-93

[32] Agar JW et al. Home haemodialysis: How it began, where it went wrong, and what it may yet be. Journal of Nephrology. 2019;**32**:331-333

[33] Barraclough KA, Agar JW. Green nephrology. Nature Reviews Nephrology. 2020;**16**(5):257-268

[34] Garcia, Sanchez JJ et al. Using chronic kidney disease as a model framework to estimate healthcare-related

environmental impact. Advances in Therapy. 2025;**42**:348-361

[35] Henderson S et al. Comparison of utilities consumption between different modalities of in-center haemodialysis: TH-PO291. Journal of the American Society of Nephrology. 2023;**34**(11S):172

[36] Chen M et al. The carbon footprints of home and in-center peritoneal dialysis in China. International Urology and Nephrology. 2017;**49**:337-343

[37] Makhloufi M et al. Haemodialysis versus peritoneal dialysis in children: An eco-audit. Nephrology Dialysis Transplantation. 2024;**39**(11):1927-1929

[38] Agar JW. Green dialysis: The environmental challenges ahead. Seminars in Dialysis. 2015;**28**(2):186-192

[39] Karkar A, Wilkie M. Peritoneal dialysis in the modern era. Peritoneal Dialysis International. 2023;**43**(4):301-314

[40] Yu X et al. Shared decision-making for a dialysis modality. Kidney International Reports. 2022;**7**(1):15-27

[41] Zawierucha J et al. Green dialysis: Let us talk about dialysis fluid. Kidney and Blood Pressure Research. 2023;**48**(1):385-391

[42] Blake PG, Diaz-Buxo JA. Adequacy of peritoneal dialysis and chronic peritoneal dialysis prescription. In: Daugirdas JT, Blake PG, Ing TS, editors. Handbook of Dialysis. 3rd ed. Philadelphia: Lippincott Williams & Wilkins; 2003. pp. 343-360

[43] Uchiyama K et al. The impact of a remote monitoring system of healthcare resource consumption in patients on automated peritoneal dialysis (APD): A simulation study. Clinical Nephrology. 2018;**90**(5):334

[44] Żebrowski P et al. Home dialysis during COVID-19 outbreak-it is worth to consider. Wiadomości Lekarskie. 2020;**73**(10):2316-2318

[45] Broadbent P et al. The public health implications of the cost-of-living crisis: Outlining mechanisms and modelling consequences. The Lancet Regional Health–Europe. 2023;**27**(April):1-8, 100585

[46] Baxter Canada. Peritoneal dialysis catalogue [Internet]. 2024 [cited 2024 Dec 23]. Available from: https://www.baxter.ca/sites/g/files/ebysai1431/files/2024-01/PD%20Catalogue%20English%20-%202024%20V.3.pdf

[47] Sorkin MI, Blake PG. Apparatus for peritoneal dialysis. In: Daugirdas JT, Blake PG, Ing TS, editors. Handbook of Dialysis. 3rd ed. Philadelphia: Lippincott Williams & Wilkins; 2003. pp. 309-332

[48] UK Kidney Association. Home dialysis utility reimbursement calculator 2022-2023 [Internet]. 2024 [cited 2024 Dec 14]. Available from: https://www.ukkidney.org/sites/renal.org/files/WKN-UKKA%20Home%20Dialysis%20Utility%20Reimbursement%20Calculator%202022-2023.xlsx

[49] Piccoli GB et al. Green nephrology and eco-dialysis: A position statement by the Italian society of nephrology. Journal of Nephrology. 2020;**33**:681-698

[50] Torreggiani M et al. Choice of the dialysis modality: Practical considerations. Journal of Clinical Medicine. 2023;**12**(9):3328

[51] Surendra NK et al. The cost of dialysis in Malaysia: Haemodialysis and continuous ambulatory peritoneal

dialysis. Malaysian Journal of Public Health Medicine. 2018;**18**(Suppl. 2):70-81

[52] Mendu ML et al. International home dialysis roundtable steering committee. Expanding utilization of home dialysis: An action agenda from the first international home dialysis roundtable. Kidney Medicine. 2021;**3**(4):635-643

[53] Ataguba JE et al. Financial protection in health revisited: Is catastrophic health spending underestimated for service-or disease-specific analysis? Health Economics. 2024;**33**(6):1229-1240

[54] McGrath A et al. Peritoneal dialysis modality choice: Not an automated decision. Clinical Journal of the American Society of Nephrology. 2024;**10**:2215

[55] NHS Wales. Kidney support welfare Wales press release [Internet]. 2023 [cited 2024 Dec 14]. Available from: https://emedia2.nhs.wales/wrcn/assets/Kidney%20News/News%202023/KSWW%20Press%20Release/Kidney%20Support%20%20Welfare%20Wales.pdf

[56] Jolliffe D, Tetteh-Baah SK. Identifying the poor–accounting for household economies of scale in global poverty estimates. World Development. 2024;**179**:106593

[57] Lopez C, Bendix J. Global Opportunity Index 2020 Focus on the GCC Countries. MPRA Paper 98513. Germany: Milken Institute, University Library of Munich; 2020

[58] World Bank. World development indicators: electricity consumption per capita (EG.USE.ELEC.KH.PC) [Internet]. 2024 [cited 2024 Dec 22]. Available from: https://databank.worldbank.org/source/world-development-indicators/Series/EG.USE.ELEC.KH.PC

[59] World Bank. Population total – Qatar, Saudi Arabia, Oman, UAE, Kuwait, Bahrain [Internet]. 2024 [cited 2024 Dec 22]. Available from: https://data.worldbank.org/indicator/SP.POP.TOTL?locations=QA-SA-OM-AE-KW-BH

[60] World Bank. Gross national income (NY.GNP) [Internet]. 2024 [cited 2024 Dec 22]. Available from: https://data.worldbank.org/indicator/NY.GNP

[61] Ashkanani AM et al. Impact of COVID-19 interventions on electricity power production: An empirical investigation in Kuwait. Electric Power Systems Research. 2022;**205**:107718

[62] Al Sahlawi M et al. Peritoneal dialysis in the Arabian gulf countries: Challenges and opportunities. Peritoneal Dialysis International. 2024;**44**(3):171-176

[63] Karam S, et al. Capacity for the management of kidney failure in the International Society of Nephrology Middle East region: Report from the 2023 ISN Global Kidney Health Atlas (ISN-GKHA). Kidney International Supplements. 1 Apr 2024;**13**(1):57-70

[64] Wang G et al. Water resource management and policy evaluation in middle eastern countries: Achieving sustainable development goal 6. Desalination and Water Treatment. 2024;**320**:100829

[65] Alsabbagh M et al. Electricity consumption in the municipal water sector in an oil-exporting, water-stressed country: The case of Bahrain. Desalination and Water Treatment. 2021;**213**:117-127

[66] Abulibdeh A. Geospatial assessment of the carbon footprint of water and electricity consumption in residential buildings in Doha, Qatar. Journal of Cleaner Production. 2024;**445**:141262

[67] Bernstein DH et al. Work-from-home, electricity, and water: Evidence from covid-19 in Qatar. Energy Strategy Reviews. 2023;**49**:101119

[68] Ibrahim AJ, Shirazi NS. Energy-water-environment nexus and the transition towards a circular economy: The case of Qatar. Circular Economy and Sustainability. 2021;**1**(April):835-850

[69] Marzooq M, Alsabbagh M, Al-Zubari W. Energy consumption in the municipal water supply sector in the Kingdom of Bahrain. Computational Water, Energy, and Environmental Engineering. 2018;**7**(03):95

[70] Abotalib M et al. The environmental life cycle assessment of different electricity options in Kuwait. Journal of Engineering Research. 2021;**9**(2):308-319

[71] Alhajeri HM et al. Energy demand in the state of Kuwait during the covid-19 pandemic: Technical, economic, and environmental perspectives. Energies. 2020;**13**(17):4370

[72] Ansari MS. The water demand management in the Kingdom of Bahrain. Journal of Engineering and Advanced Technology. 2013;**2**(5):544-554

[73] Hajjaj ME, Hashim AH. Water security and stability in the Kingdom of Bahrain. Desalination and Water Treatment. 2013;**51**(1-3):67-74

[74] Al-Noaimi MA. Development of water information system for the Kingdom of Bahrain. Desalination and Water Treatment. 2022;**263**(July):267-281

[75] Abulibdeh A. Spatiotemporal analysis of water-electricity consumption in the context of the COVID-19 pandemic across six socioeconomic sectors in Doha City, Qatar. Applied Energy. 2021;**304**:117864

[76] Lawler J et al. The domestic water sector in Qatar. In: Sustainable Qatar: Social, Political and Environmental Perspectives. Singapore: Springer Nature; 2022. pp. 193-209

[77] Al-Shueili AA. Financial sustainability of the water sector in the Sultanate of Oman (Doctoral dissertation). Loughborough University

[78] Gastli A et al. GIS-based assessment of combined CSP electric power and seawater desalination plant for Duqum—Oman. Renewable and Sustainable Energy Reviews. 2010;**14**(2):821-827

[79] Hadi K. Current status, challenges, and future management strategies for water resources of Kuwait. In: Terrestrial Environment and Ecosystems of Kuwait: Assessment and Restoration. Cham: Springer Nature Switzerland; 2024. pp. 141-169

[80] Alzaabi MS, Mezher T. Analyzing existing UAE national water, energy and food nexus related strategies. Renewable and Sustainable Energy Reviews. 2021;**144**:111031

[81] Almulhim AI, Aina YA. Understanding household water-use behavior and consumption patterns during COVID-19 lockdown in Saudi Arabia. Water. 2022;**14**(3):314

[82] Al-Saidi M, Saliba S. Water, energy and food supply security in the Gulf cooperation council (GCC) countries—A risk perspective. Water. 2019;**11**(3):455

[83] Ali SM, Acquaye A. An examination of water-energy-food nexus: From theory to application. Renewable and Sustainable Energy Reviews. 2024;**202**:114669

[84] Elbalki M et al. Optimizing integrated water and electrical networks through a holistic water–energy nexus approach. Sustainability. 2024;**16**(9):3783

[85] International Monetary Fund. Middle East and Central Asia Dept. "Gulf Cooperation Council: Pursuing Visions Amid Geopolitical Turbulence: Economic Prospects and Policy Challenges for the GCC Countries", Policy Papers 2024, 066 (2024). 10.5089/9798400295744.007 [Accessed: December 23, 2024]

[86] United Nations Convention to Combat Desertification (UNCCD). COP 16 [Internet]. 2024 [cited 2024 Dec 22]. Available from: https://www.unccd.int/cop16

[87] COP28. Official COP28 website [Internet]. 2024 [cited 2024 Dec 22]. Available from: https://www.cop28.com/en/

[88] Al-Omar HA et al. Value drivers for pharmaceutical products in health technology assessment (HTA) in Saudi Arabia: Results from a capacity building, multi-stakeholder workshop. Saudi Pharmaceutical Journal. 2021;**29**(9):946-954

[89] Alkhamis A, Miraj SA. Access to health care in Saudi Arabia: Development in the context of vision 2030. In: Handbook of Healthcare in the Arab World. Cham: Springer International Publishing; 2021. pp. 1629-1660

[90] Asmri MA et al. The public health care system and primary care services in Saudi Arabia: A system in transition. Eastern Mediterranean Health Journal. 2020;**26**(4):468-476

[91] Al-Aqeel S. Health technology assessment in Saudi Arabia. Expert Review of Pharmacoeconomics & Outcomes Research. 2018;**18**(4):393-402

[92] Al-Hanawi MK. The healthcare system in Saudi Arabia: How can we best move forward with funding to protect equitable and accessible care for all. International Journal of Healthcare. 2017;**3**(2):78-94

[93] Alkhamis A et al. Financing healthcare in gulf cooperation council countries: A focus on Saudi Arabia. The International Journal of Health Planning and Management. 2014;**29**(1):e64-e82

[94] Ahmed G et al. Strategic leadership and economic transformation: The United Arab Emirates (UAE) model. Journal of Global Business Research and Practice. 2024;**1**(1):1-18

[95] Qureshi W. The role of human Capital in the Implementation of healthcare innovation in the UAE. In: Human Capital in the Middle East: A UAE Perspective. Cham: Palgrave Macmillan, Switzerland; 2020. pp. 275-310

[96] Alshamari S. The Qatar health system: Challenges and opportunities. Network Intelligence Studies. 2017;**5**(9):47-56

[97] AlSajari MM. Facilities management in hospitals: A comparison of the United States and Kuwait. (Doctoral dissertation). University of Miami

[98] Al Mawali AH et al. Oman vision 2050 for health research: A strategic plan for the future based on the past and present experience. Oman Medical Journal. 2017;**32**(2):86

[99] Al Arrayed A et al. Renal transplant is an established and successful treatment for end-stage renal failure in Bahrain. Bahrain Medical Bulletin. 2000;**22**:60-63

[100] Mehdi I et al. General oncology care in Oman. In: Cancer in the Arab World. Singapore: Springer Singapore; 2022. pp. 175-193

[101] Aljelban AS et al. Assessment of accountable care organization strategies: A qualitative approach. Open Journal of Business and Management. 2024;**12**(01):1-7

[102] Hamad A et al. Overview of procurement and reimbursement of Pharmaceuticals in Saudi Arabia, United Arab Emirates, Qatar, and Egypt: Challenges and opportunities. Global Journal on Quality and Safety in Healthcare. 2023;**6**(4):127-136

[103] Alnashmi M et al. Evaluating service satisfaction and sustainability of the Afya insurance scheme in Kuwait: An exploratory analysis. Clinico Economics and Outcomes Research. 2024;**16**(August):597-617

[104] AlSahow A et al. Demographics and key clinical characteristics of hemodialysis patients from the Gulf cooperation council countries enrolled in the dialysis outcomes and practice patterns study phase 5 (2012-2015). Saudi Journal of Kidney Diseases and Transplantation. 2016;**27**(Suppl. 1):S12-S23

[105] Esteve A et al. A global perspective on household size and composition, 1970-2020. Genus. 2024;**80**(1):2

[106] Al-Za'abi R et al. Sun-202 epidemiology of end stage renal disease (ESRD) of Oman since 1983 to 2018: A secondary data analysis study. Kidney International Reports. 2020;**5**(3):S283-S284

[107] Aljenaidi H et al. Quality of life in hemodialysis versus peritoneal dialysis patients in Bahrain. Cureus. 2023;**15**(11):1-11, e49408

[108] Al Malki H et al. Renal replacement therapy in Qatar—Past, present and future. Open Journal of Nephrology. 2018;**8**(2):42-55

[109] Al Agha R et al. Current state of vascular access in patients on hemodialysis in Bahrain. Journal of the Bahrain Medical Society. 2021;**33**(1):26-30

[110] Saudi Electricity Company. Consumption tariffs [Internet]. 2024 [cited 2024 Dec 22]. Available from: https://www.se.com.sa/en/Ourservices/ColumnC/Bills-and-Consumption/ConsumptionTariffs

[111] Marafiq. Power tariff [Internet]. 2024 [cited 2024 Dec 22]. Available from: https://www.marafiq.com.sa/en/partnering-with-us/power-tariff/

[112] Electricity and Water Authority (EWA), Bahrain. Electricity and water tariffs [Internet]. 2024 [cited 2024 Dec 15]. Available from: https://www.ewa.bh/en/Customer/BillsTariffs/electricitywater-tariffs

[113] Kahramaa, Qatar. Tariff [Internet]. 2024 [cited 2024 Dec 15]. Available from: https://www.km.qa/CustomerService/Pages/Tariff.aspx

[114] APSRC, Oman. Tariffs [Internet]. 2024 [cited 2024 Dec 14]. Available from: https://www.apsr.om/en/tariffs

[115] Ministry of Electricity and Water, Kuwait. Tariff page [Internet]. 2024 [cited 2024 Dec 22]. Available from: https://smportal.mew.gov.kw/msdpweb/primary/_-iZnyIUmX

[116] Dubai Electricity and Water Authority (DEWA). Tariff calculator [Internet]. 2024 [cited 2024 Dec 15]. Available from: https://www.dewa.gov.ae/en/consumer/billing/tariffcalculator

[117] Dubai Electricity and Water Authority (DEWA). Slab tariff [Internet]. 2024 [cited 2024 Dec 15]. Available from: https://www.dewa.gov.ae/en/consumer/billing/slab-tariff

[118] XE.com. Currency converter [Internet]. 2024 [cited 2024 Dec 15]. Available from: www.xe.com

[119] Brown EA et al. International Society for Peritoneal Dialysis practice recommendations: Prescribing high-quality goal-directed peritoneal dialysis. Peritoneal Dialysis International. 2020;**40**(3):244-253

[120] Walker RC et al. Home hemodialysis: A comprehensive review of patient-centered and economic considerations. ClinicoEconomics and Outcomes Research. 2017;**9**(February):149-161

[121] Marafiq. Water tariff [Internet]. 2024 [cited 2024 Dec 22]. Available from: https://www.marafiq.com.sa/en/partnering-with-us/water-tariff/

[122] Almulhim AI et al. A segmentation approach to understanding water consumption behavioral patterns among households in Saudi Arabia for a sustainable future. Resources, Environment and Sustainability. 2024;**15**:100144

[123] Amir N et al. A working partnership: A review of shared decision-making in nephrology. Nephrology. 2021;**26**(11):851-857

[124] Finderup J et al. Evaluation of a shared decision-making intervention for dialysis choice at four Danish hospitals: A qualitative study of patient perspective. BMJ Open. 2019;**9**(10):e029090

[125] Dahlerus C et al. Patient perspectives on the choice of dialysis modality: Results from the empowering patients on choices for renal replacement therapy (EPOCH-RRT) study. American Journal of Kidney Diseases. 2016;**68**(6):901-910

[126] Walker RC et al. Patients' and caregivers' expectations and experiences of remote monitoring for peritoneal dialysis: A qualitative interview study. Peritoneal Dialysis International. 2020;**40**(6):540-547

[127] International Energy Agency (IEA). Oman [Internet]. 2024 [cited 2024 Dec 22]. Available from: https://www.iea.org/countries/oman

[128] International Energy Agency (IEA). Bahrain [Internet]. 2024 [cited 2024 Dec 22]. Available from: https://www.iea.org/countries/bahrain

[129] International Energy Agency (IEA). Kuwait [Internet]. 2024 [cited 2024 Dec 22]. Available from: https://www.iea.org/countries/kuwait

[130] International Energy Agency (IEA). Qatar [Internet]. 2024 [cited 2024 Dec 22]. Available from: https://www.iea.org/countries/qatar

[131] International Energy Agency (IEA). United Arab Emirates [Internet]. 2024 [cited 2024 Dec 22]. Available from: https://www.iea.org/countries/united-arab-emirates

[132] International Energy Agency (IEA). Saudi Arabia [Internet]. 2024 [cited 2024 Dec 22]. Available from: https://www.iea.org/countries/saudi-arabia

[133] International Energy Agency (IEA). Australia [Internet]. 2024 [cited 2024 Dec 22]. Available from: https://www.iea.org/countries/australia

[134] International Energy Agency (IEA). China [Internet]. 2024 [cited 2024 Dec 22]. Available from: https://www.iea.org/countries/china

Chapter 5

Peritoneal Dialysis in Children

Souad Chelghoum, Salah-eddine Benfarhi and Atmane Seba

Abstract

For children undergoing chronic dialysis, peritoneal dialysis (PD) is still the most popular method, especially for younger patients and those living in lower- and middle-income nations (LMICs). When compared to extracorporeal therapy, PD for acute kidney injury (AKI) in children has a lengthy history of success. It is still widely utilized, particularly in Europe, in both high- and low-resource environments. The use of PD for AKI in low birthweight and post-cardiac surgery neonates is of special interest in these areas. There are few high-quality randomized trials conducted on children, and most of the data used in clinical practice today are either taken from observational cohort studies on children or extrapolated from studies conducted on adults. Guidelines for starting dialysis, choosing a modality, clearing tiny solutes, maintaining kidney function, and removing fluid from children receiving post-natal dialysis are provided by the International Society for Peritoneal Dialysis (ISPD). The evidence for PD in children is still quite weak, The recommendation's strength and level of evidence are GRADE-ed. Although every patient should still aim for optimal dialysis, it is crucial to have a thorough conversation about expectations for dialysis with caregivers and patients who are fully informed.

Keywords: chronic peritoneal dialysis, acute kidney injury, ISPD, children, optimal dialysis

1. Introduction

1.1 Chronic peritoneal dialysis

Since peritoneal dialysis (PD) may be applied practically anywhere, it is very affordable and offers the benefits of a home-based treatment, which is the most popular chronic dialysis modality in children, especially for younger children, and in lower- and middle-income countries (LMICs) [1]. The main factors contributing to better survival and results include technological advancements in dialysis, enhanced dialysis fluids, and clinical know-how in the treatment of problems associated with dialysis [2]. Still, there are not many excellent prospective studies or even randomized controlled trials (RCTs) including children with PD.

While providing a broader view of the numerous difficulties confronted by that individual, the International Society for Peritoneal Dialysis (ISPD) publications [3–5] highlights the need for a person-centered approach with shared decision making between the clinical care team and the person doing peritoneal dialysis. A review of the literature allowed recommendations to be released for the pediatric peritoneal dialysis. A recommendation of grade 1 is strongly advised, but one of grade 2 is not. The suggestions' level of evidence is indicated by the letters (A through D).

2. Peritoneal dialysis practice in children

Children on maintenance PD continue to present challenges in accurately assessing their volume status. To differentiate weight increases attributed to volume overload from physiological changes associated with growth, routine and frequent assessment is necessary. In pediatric dialysis patients, hypertension is mostly volume-related, although it can also have other contributing factors. In a prospective longitudinal study, Karava et al. measure serum albumin, blood pressure, and bioimpedance spectroscopy (BIS) at various intervals over a 6-month period in children with a median age of 12.6 years. They illustrate how BIS is superior to weight or blood pressure monitoring for determining volume status [6]. When evaluating serial changes in the relative overhydration status as opposed to a single measure, BIS was especially helpful. These findings corroborate more extensive pediatric research that suggests routine multimodal hydration status assessments, including the use of objective metrics like BIS [2, 7, 8]. Comparatively, BIS-guided fluid management did not show an additional benefit to achieve euvolemia and did not affect the decline in RKF in non-anuric PD adult patients [9, 10].

It is not always fair to extrapolate research findings on adult PD to the pediatric population. Hennessy et al., for instance, address dosage recommendations for intraperitoneal vancomycin based on pharmacokinetic modeling in this issue of PD [11]. They note that the dose guidelines currently in use, which are based on adult practice, may cause vancomycin toxicity in children [12]. Even though a lot has been accomplished, the field of pediatric nephrology still has a ways to go before offering children high-quality PD that is supported by evidence-based practice. Because pediatric maintenance dialysis is so uncommon, the numerous unanswered concerns about the best treatment approaches for children and how they affect clinical outcomes can only be addressed by large-scale, international research or registries.

The granular data collected by the International Pediatric Peritoneal Dialysis Network registry [13] on many elements of dialysis therapy have significantly enhanced our comprehension of the potential hazards, results, and approaches to treating pediatric PD. Similar to this, quality improvement programs like The Standardizing Care to Improve Outcomes in Pediatric End Stage Renal Disease collaborative [14] have found modifiable risk factors and practices that affect common complications of PD. These initiatives use large-scale collaboration to identify and promote effective interventions across pediatric care settings.

More RCTs and well-conducted multicenter registry-based observational studies are needed to conduct studies in pediatric PD. These studies can be highly efficient and cost-effective while producing crucial evidence that is unique to children with PD.

2.1 Start of dialysis

We recommend starting dialysis in children with an estimated glomerular filtration rate (eGFR) of less than 10 ml/ml/1.73 m^2 or when the child develops uremic symptoms that are not responsive to treatment with medication or dietary changes (*Level of evidence—Grade 2D*) [2, 4].

Rationale: The decision about when to start dialysis is complicated and should take into account the eGFR as well as signs and symptoms of uremia, which include:

- declining weight and/or height centiles; growth failure;
- inability to maintain euvolemia with the development of hypertension and/or significant peripheral edema;
- deterioration in nutritional status; and
- subjective complaints from the patient, such as nausea, fatigue, loss of appetite, and a perceived low quality of life.

These problems must be demonstrated to be persistent and unresponsive to dietary and/or pharmacological control before dialysis is started. The length of time that uremic symptoms persist before dialysis is considered essential will depend on how severe they are and how much discomfort they are causing the youngster. When a child is old enough, their caretakers and their medical professionals should have a conversation before deciding to begin dialysis. From 16.5% in 1995 to 40.8% in 2015, the proportion of pediatric patients in the US who started dialysis with an eGFR greater than 10 ml/min/1.73 m^2 has increased.

A recent review of data from the United States Renal Data System (USRDS) revealed that 29% (4481) of the 15,473 children who started dialysis between 1995 and 2015 did so while their eGFR was greater than 10 ml/min/1.73 m^2 (median 12.8 ml/min/1.73 m^2) [15]. Patients who started dialysis at a higher eGFR had a 24% higher risk of death (censored at kidney transplant) than patients whose eGFR was <10 ml/min/1.73 m^2 (median eGFR 6.5 ml/min/1.73 m^2). Nevertheless, for the PD population (n = 6148), the higher risk of mortality linked to "early" dialysis initiation did not reach statistical significance when dialysis mode was taken into account [15].

About 2963 children from 21 different countries had their dialysis initiations investigated in a new registry report from the European Society of Pediatric Nephrology/European Renal Association-European Dialysis and Transplant Association Registry [16]. Regarding mortality, growth, or access to transplantation, there were no clinically significant advantages observed for individuals who began dialysis at an eGFR of more than or less than 8 mL/min/1.73 m^2. However, hypertension was more common in late initiators [16]. When choosing whether to start or stop dialysis in children with ESKD, the presence of cardiovascular risk factors, such as high blood pressure, should be considered as this impacts the survival rate.

The accuracy of eGFR estimation in late stages of CKD must also be interpreted cautiously, even if these studies are registry reports only and should be treated with caution [17].

The Schwartz bedside formula, which was created for the CKD in children study, is most accurate when applied to children with GFRs between 15 and 75 ml/min/1.73 m^2 and when standardized serum creatinine methods traceable to the isotope dilution mass spectrometry technique are used [16]. If a measured GFR is available, it may be helpful in situations where a creatinine-based estimate may be erroneous (such as in patients with low muscle mass) and where there is poor agreement between the Schwartz bedside calculation and a univariate cystatin C-based model. Equations based on blood creatinine and cystatin C readings together yield a more accurate prediction in individuals, both young and old, than equations based on only one biomarker [18, 19].

2.2 Choose your modality

When choosing a dialysis modality for a child, considerations such as the age and size, any comorbidities, the availability of family support, modality contraindications, the dialysis team's experience, and the child's and parents'/caregivers' preference should all be taken into account. When choosing the best dialysis modality for a child, it is important to take into account the preservation of dialysis access, both peritoneal and vascular (*Level of evidence—Ungraded*) [2, 5].

Rationale: Studies have not been conducted to determine which treatment is better for children with end-stage kidney disease (ESKD)—hemodialysis (HD) or PD [20]. The contraindications for the use of peritoneal dialysis (PD) in children are seen in table [1]. International registries indicate that PD is the most popular and preferable modality for younger children (the USRDS lists children under 9 years old, the UK renal replacement registry lists children under 5 years old, and the European Society for Pediatric Nephrology registry lists children under 9 years old) [21]. Actually, according to statistics from the USRDS, 64% of patients weighing less than 20 kg had PD as their first renal replacement therapy between 1996 and 2015, compared to only 31.8% of patients weighing between 20 and 50 kg. For very small patients, for whom maintaining a functional and complication-free vascular access might be challenging, PD is especially beneficial.

In cooperation with the ESPN/ERA-EDTA Registry, the Australian and New Zealand Dialysis and Transplantation Registry, and the Japanese Society for Dialysis Therapy Registry, the IPPN published data on the outcomes and survival of 264 patients who began chronic dialysis during the neonatal period in 2014 [22]. These people had survival rates of 81 and 76% at 2 and 5 years, respectively. Neurologic illness was the largest risk factor for mortality. These results showed that CPD that began in the neonatal period can be successfully treated, despite severe therapeutic challenges associated with comorbidities, infections, malnourishment, hypertension, and development failure.

Home dialysis treatments, such as PD using an automated PD (APD) cycling device, help school-age children attend class regularly. When using anticoagulation is contraindicated or in children with cardiovascular instability, PD is also favored over HD. While PD should not be viewed as the "default option," families should be counseled on the various dialysis modalities available while taking into account their proximity to a pediatric HD center and their capacity to establish and maintain a proper vascular access. In LMICs, the use of PD has grown among both adults and children [23]. Crucially, after completely educating the child and family on the options available and medically suitable, the choice of dialysis modality needs to be carefully considered. Respecting the child's and parents'/caregivers' choice should occur whenever it is feasible and not detrimental.

Changes in dwell time have an effect on purification as well as ultrafiltration (UF). While a brief stay preferentially eliminates tiny solutes like urea, it also benefits UF. Due to the time-dependent decrease of the crystalloid osmotic gradient, a prolonged stay is beneficial for both peritoneal fluid reabsorption and the elimination of uremic toxins. Specifically, prolonged daytime stays in APD may lead to notable reabsorption of water and sodium; in these situations, icodextrin may be of consideration. Because of the increased volume of diffusion and the recruitment of peritoneal surface area, increasing dwell volume facilitates the removal of solutes like sodium. However, very high intraperitoneal pressure (IPP) combined with a very large fill volume may cause back-filtration, which lowers salt and UF clearance. These ideas, along with the distinct transport and pressure kinetics discovered from IPP measurements and peritoneal equilibration studies, lead us to propose mixing long stays and a large fill volume with short durations to promote UF and solute evacuation. This idea is supported by the findings of a recent randomized cross-over experiment as well as past observational data in children: solute removal and blood pressure improved, and the absolute UF and UF in relation to the supplied glucose increased [24].

Of course, it is impossible to overstate how important it is to acknowledge the care burden that this home-based dialysis therapy places on families. Apart from the dialysis process itself, there are other burdens such as choosing the right PD solution each day, worrying about potential complications, including peritonitis, having trouble relieving patient drain discomfort, and handling machine problems securely. As part of the modality selection process, families need to be fully informed about the care burden associated with doing physical therapy so that suitable support networks may be established.

This procedure would benefit from a formal evaluation of the patient's and caregiver's quality of life perceptions [25, 26]. In certain countries, "Assisted PD," in which a qualified dialysis technician regularly comes to the patient's house to set up the PD machine and/or connect and detach the child from PD, is provided. This approach increases the number of patients who can undergo PD by giving families the necessary support (**Table 1**).

There is a lack of extensive pediatric research demonstrating a relationship between patient outcome and residual kidney function (RKF) in children with PD. Even though the mean total solute clearance of the two patient groups was similar, a single-center observation of a juvenile PD population revealed that children with RKF had superior growth velocity compared to children without RKF [27]. RKF may therefore be beneficial for both growth and the accomplishment of solute clearance objectives [28, 29]. Furthermore, there is evidence that children receiving PD therapy lose RKF more slowly than those receiving HD therapy [30, 31].

2.3 Peritoneal access

A functioning peritoneal dialysis catheter (PDC) is necessary for successful PD. Catheter type, exit site orientation, placement technique, timing of initial catheter use, and exit site care are some of the factors that may have an impact on catheter performance. Ideally, there should be minimal mechanical or infectious issues as a result of the placement method, the PD catheter's features, and the catheter's maintenance. There are several ways to install PD catheters, including surgical, laparoscopic/peritoneoscopic, blind or Seldinger, and fluoroscopic methods; however, the success of each method varies in terms of catheter survival and complication rates. Nephrologists prefer peritoneoscopic and fluoroscopic procedures because they are less intrusive, employ local anesthetic, can be completed reasonably easily in an ambulatory setting, are less expensive, and do not have the same mortality risks as general anesthesia [32–34]. This research emphasizes the benefits of nephrologists inserting catheters and concentrates on peritoneoscopic and fluoroscopic procedures.

Absolute contraindications	Relative contraindications
Defects of the abdominal wall, such as gastroschisis and omphalocele	The existence of colostomies and ileostomies
Bladder exstrophy	Newborns with severe organomegaly
Diaphragmatic hernia	Inadequate housing for receiving dialysis at home
Destroyed the peritoneum	Inadequate assistance for caregivers
Failing peritoneal membrane	Imminent or recently completed major abdominal surgery
Open abdomen	Paralytic ileus
Abdominal compartment syndrome	Open chest following cardiac surgery
Fungal peritonitis	Difficulty breathing for the patient
	Pleuroperitoneal connection allowing dialysate in the chest
	Inguinal hernia
	Hypercatabolic renal failure where clearance of small solutes may be insufficient
	Situations where exact removal of large volumes of fluid is required
	Abdominal wall cellulitis or abdominal wall burn

Table 1.
Contraindications for the use of DP in children.

2.3.1 Peritoneoscopic insertion of a PD catheter

As a result, the intraperitoneal structures can be directly seen thanks to the peritoneoscopic approach. Nephrologists are the ones who employ this procedure the most frequently, and their use is growing quickly [35]. A device to advance the cuff into the musculature, a much smaller scope and puncture size, only one peritoneal puncture site, air insufflated into the peritoneum instead of CO_2, and local anesthesia (conscious sedation is used in some centers) as opposed to general anesthesia are some of the ways that peritoneoscopic placement differs from laparoscopic techniques [35].

2.3.2 PD catheter insertion using fluoroscopic technique

Unlike peritoneoscopic insertion, this method necessitates the use of a fluoroscope [33, 34]. Similar to peritoneoscopy, this operation can be carried out in an ambulatory setting with conscious sedation, and patients can typically resume eating right away following the procedure [33, 34].

Marking the upper border of the deep cuff on the abdomen 2 to 3 cm lateral to the midline and aligning the upper border of the PD catheter coil with the superior edge of the pubic symphysis establishes the insertion site. This will make it more probable that the catheter will rest on the pelvic floor.

2.3.3 Catheter's types

The majority of PD access devices used worldwide are made up of the basic double Dacron (polyester) cuff, straight and coiled-tip Tenckhoff catheters, and their swan neck versions with an arc bend completed in the intercuff section. The fundamental Tenckhoff catheter designs have undergone a number of changes in order to address the frequent mechanical issues of tissue adhesion, tip movement, and pericatheter leakage [36]. There does not seem to be a better catheter than the conventional Tenckhoff catheter with two cuffs. In order to decrease peritonitis and increase catheter survival duration, double cuff catheters are advised. The ideal peritoneal entrance point is paramedian or lateral. The exit point ought to face downhill or to the side. In general, upward-directed exit sites ought to be avoided [3].

2.3.4 Prophylactic antibiotics

Strict sterile technique is required to prevent colonization of the Tenckhoff catheter and/or contamination during insertion, as these events raise the risk of future peritonitis. Prophylactic antibiotics, when administered in conjunction with sterile procedure, reduce the incidence of peritonitis; nevertheless, they do not always prevent infections if sterile technique is not followed. It is recommended to abide by the guidelines for the use of this medication for chronic PD catheter placement in the lack of data regarding the use of prophylactic antibiotics in the setting of acute PD [12]. The choice of antibiotic depends on availability, procedure schedule, and local bacterial susceptibilities. It is widely acknowledged that gram-positive organisms are the most crucial to defend against. According to the ISPD pediatric guidelines, prophylactic antibiotics should be administered no later than 60 minutes before PD catheter insertion in order to ensure sufficient tissue levels before the initial incision.

2.3.5 Manual PD delivery systems

In chronic patients, closed systems are linked to lower rates of peritonitis when compared to normal spiking systems.

2.3.6 Automated PD systems

In the 1980s, APD using a cycling device was put into clinical practice. It effectively controlled electrolyte and metabolism in ESKD patients while also reducing the incidence of peritonitis [37, 38].

2.3.7 Complications in CPD

2.3.7.1 Leakage

The most frequent problem is leakage, which has been documented to occur up to 12.8% of the time [39]. After a patient is able to walk, dialysis leakage usually becomes more noticeable and happens in the first few weeks or months following catheter implantation. According to convention, a leak is considered early if it happens within 30 days of the catheter being inserted and late if it happens after that time. Dialysate leaks can occur more frequently in babies, albeit this depends on the definition [40].

2.3.7.2 Bleeding

While bleeding is a common consequence during PD catheter implantation, about 1–5% of surgeries result in serious bleeding [41].

2.3.7.3 Visceral injury

During the catheter placement operation, it is possible for the small or large bowel and bladder to sustain unintentional injuries. Injury frequently happens when the PD catheter is advanced into the lower abdomen using a stylet or during entrance into the abdominal cavity.

2.3.7.4 Dysfunction of mechanical flow

A primary reason of PD catheter malfunction is mechanical issues, which show up as insufficient dialysate input and/or outflow. It makes sense to follow the dialysate flow channel to identify the causes of mechanical failure [42].

2.3.7.5 Peritonitis

The pediatric chronic PD guidelines should be followed in order to diagnose, prevent, and treat acute peritonitis [12]. Infections did not become the main cause of access failure until after the first year of PD. It was not possible to ascertain if the administration of preventive antibiotics at the exit site over time had any impact on the frequency of infection-related access revisions in our sample. In contrast to simultaneous removal and placement in the event of relapsing peritonitis, the ISPD pediatric consensus guidelines recommend a two-stage catheter removal and reinsertion in patients diagnosed with fungal, enteral, or refractory peritonitis [12].

2.4 Cardiovascular disease, blood pressure, and level of hydration

2.4.1 Evaluation of the state of hydration

In order to help guide the PD prescription and ultrafiltration requirements, we suggest evaluating the patient's dry weight at each clinic visit with clinical evaluation, including weight and blood pressure (BP) measurement, laboratory parameters, and objective measurements of fluid status using bioimpedance spectroscopy, where available *(Level of evidence—Grade 2C)* [2, 43].

Rationale: Cardiovascular disease continues to be the leading cause of death for children receiving dialysis, making up 30% of all fatalities [44]. The presence of hypertension, prolonged fluid overload, altered mineral metabolism, and inflammation are the strongest predictors. These factors collectively result in left ventricular hypertrophy (LVH), which is an intermediate end point of cardiovascular morbidity in patients with CKD/ESKD and an independent risk factor [43, 45].

The approach most commonly employed to determine a patient's level of hydration is clinical examination. To evaluate the fluid status of patients on PD, physical examination for edema, blood pressure monitoring, and laboratory markers including hemoglobin/hematocrit and serum albumin levels are frequently employed. A hypervolemic state may be indicated by the existence of erythropoietin-stimulating agent (ESA)-resistant anemia. A higher prevalence of hypertension, left ventricular hypertrophy, and hypoalbuminemia—all of which are probably caused by hypervolemia—correlated with anemia that was poorly responsive to ESAs in a study on the management of anemia in over 1400 children conducted by the International Pediatric Peritoneal Dialysis Network (IPPN) [46]. Even though more than 90% of patients received prescriptions for ESAs, one-fourth of the children had hemoglobin (HB) levels that were below target [46].

The necessity for adequate cognitive functioning at school, the need for regular physical activity, and the requirement to restrict exposure to blood products in order to maximize the possibility of transplantation make optimal anemia treatment especially critical for juvenile ESKD patients [47].

Blood pressure and volume status were the most significant drivers in a later IPPN research evaluating risk variables for LVH [34]. According to Bakkaloglu et al., children with systolic hypertension had a more than twofold increased incidence of LVH. When compared to children whose LVH regressed or who had normal LV shape, children who developed or had persistent LVH had systolic office blood pressure that was 7 mm higher. The fact that some individuals showed regression of LVH raises the possibility that the myocardium is somewhat malleable and can be better shaped with better therapeutic care. Concentric geometry was shown to be protected against by high total fluid output (sum of urine and PD-related ultrafiltration), while patients undergoing automated PD (which has a higher fluid removal capacity than CAPD) appeared to be somewhat protected.

Bioimpedance spectroscopy (BIS), measurement of circulating natriuretic peptide, lung ultrasonography for extravascular lung water or lung B lines, inferior vena cava diameter and its collapsing index, and heavy water dilution studies are additional techniques to assess the fluid status of the PD patient. There is, however, a dearth of information regarding the application of these techniques in juveniles. BIS was proposed as an objective way to measure hydration status in children receiving dialysis (PD and HD) in a prospective, observational research [8].

The BIS determined weight in this study showed a strong correlation with higher levels of N-terminal pro-brain natriuretic peptide, left ventricular end-diastolic diameter, and peripheral pulse pressure, while the clinical assessment of "dry weight" showed poor correlation with this determined weight. The study also observed a significant disparity between hydration status and blood pressure, indicating that variables other than volume overload might be responsible for elevated blood pressure in certain dialysis patients [8]. It should be remembered that hypoalbuminemia and muscular atrophy can also cause tissues to become overhydrated.

2.5 Controlling the level of hydration

We propose as a means of achieving euvolemia and normotension in the child with PD:

- dietary sodium and fluid restriction;

- encouraging the use of RAS inhibitors and promoting residual diuresis (with careful monitoring for hyperkalemia and temporary withdrawal during episodes of dehydration);

- evaluation of the peritoneal membrane transport capacity with the peritoneal equilibration test (PET) can help with the modification of the dialysis prescription, changing the fill volume, dwell time, and/or dialysate dextrose concentration. Repeating the PET should be taken into consideration in individuals who are suspected of having changed peritoneal membrane transport characteristics during the course of CPD (practice points);

- icodextrin is used to improve ultrafiltration *(Level of evidence—Grade 2D)* [2, 3].

Rationale: To reach or maintain euvolemia and a normal blood pressure, the majority of children with PD will need to follow dietary sodium and fluid restrictions. When imposing salt restriction on children with high RKF and/or sodium losses owing to dialysis, care should be taken because depleting salt might cause hypotension and stunted growth. On rare occasions, serious side effects such as anterior ischemic optic atrophy and blindness may potentially follow [48]. The Kidney Disease Improving Global Outcomes (KDIGO) Clinical Practice Guideline for BP management in CKD, the Clinical Practice Guideline for Screening and Management of High Blood Pressure in Children and Adolescents, and the Kidney Disease Outcomes Quality Initiative (KDOQI) Clinical Practice Guideline for Nutrition in Children with CKD all contain pediatric-specific recommendations regarding salt and fluid management that should be followed to help guide salt and water management [22, 49, 50].

For the majority of patients, the PD prescription is made to maximize fluid evacuation [51]. The lowest dialysate dextrose concentration necessary to produce the requisite ultrafiltration volume should be included in the prescription. Because they may induce damage to the peritoneal membrane and jeopardize or prevent long-term membrane function for dialysis, hypertonic solutions should be avoided. When increased ultrafiltration is sought without exposing the peritoneal membrane to PD solutions with a high dextrose content, other PD solutions, such as those that use icodextrin as the osmotic agent, should be taken into consideration [52].

Specifically, icodextrin improves the long-dwell ultrafiltration volume in high and high-average transporters and inhanses phosphate clearance. It is noteworthy that icodextrin reabsorption can happen and that younger children [53] do not benefit from it as much as older children and adults do. The dialysate fill volume employed may have an impact on the efficacy [52]. In children exhibiting hypertension or volume overload, it is generally recommended to aim for positive ultrafiltration during all daytime or nighttime interactions. To optimize solute clearance and ultrafiltration volume, the drain volume specifically needs to be positive following the nighttime dwell of continuous ambulatory PD and the daytime dwell(s) of continuous cyclic PD (CCPD). In the IPPN cohort, the effect of the APD prescription on daily ultrafiltration volume was evaluated. A mean daily UF volume of 600 + 680 ml/m2 was obtained from over 2500 youngsters and over 7800 observations. The average dextrose concentration (240 ml more UF per percentage increase in glucose concentration), the number of cycles, and the fill volumes during the day and at night, all directly and significantly affected the ultrafiltration volume after adjusting for age, time on PD, and RKF; contrary to, the UF was inversely associated with the dwell time (34 ml less UF per hour increase; $p < 0.001$) [54].

As previously mentioned, the PET results should be used to guide the adjustment of the dialysis dwell duration in order to maximize ultrafiltration. Patients who may have altered peritoneal membrane transport characteristics (e.g., history of peritonitis and long-term use of hypertonic PD solutions) may benefit most from a revision of the PET. Aiming at a fill volume of 600–800 ml/m^2 body surface area (BSA) in children under the age of two and 1100–1400 ml/m^2 BSA in older children, the fill volumes should also be optimized whenever possible [24]. It is advised to gradually increase the volume as the patient is able. In certain situations, the intraperitoneal pressure (IPP) may be measured in order to help prescribe the fill volume without going above a safe IPP.

For the majority of children, a safe IPP limit is thought to be an upper limit of about 14 cm of H_2O or a mean fill volume of 1400 ml/m^2 [24]. A typical problem that can be avoided with careful laxative use is an increase in IPP due to severe constipation. It is crucial to take precautions to prevent clinical overfill and a high IPP since they might lead to emesis, poor ultrafiltration due to increased lymphatic absorption, and hernia formation.

Using an automated PD software that has been modified, it could be feasible to optimize sodium and fluid management and encourage small pore transport by changing the PD prescription. Sequential short- and longer-dwell exchanges with small and large dwell volumes, respectively, are employed in modified automated PD [55]. Further prospective crossover trials in adults and children are necessary for validation. A crossover trial in adults and a pilot research in children indicate that salt and fluid elimination are increased by adapted automated PD, leading to improved BP control when compared with conventional PD.

It is best to keep people with RKF away from aminoglycosides and other nephrotoxic medications. Controlling the hydration status requires swiftly resolving insults (such infection and dehydration) that might cause acute kidney injury (AKI) and impaired diuresis. About 401 pediatric patients in the IPPN registry who started PD with significant daily residual diuresis ($\geq$ 100 ml/m^2/BSA) had their urine output prospectively tracked by Ha et al. [44]. Children with glomerular dysfunction, reduced urine output at the onset of Parkinson's disease (PD), high ultrafiltration volume, and usage of icodextrin experienced a much faster decline in daily urine volume.

Using diuretics to increase the amount of salt and water excreted in the urine is also something to think about. In order to achieve euvolemia in patients with RKF, the use of diuretics may be preferable over raising the dialysate dextrose content because hypertonic solutions may cause damage to the peritoneal membrane. Since icodextrin-based therapies could not be available in LMICs, the usage of diuretics may also be very advantageous in these settings. Those who received diuretics had an 80% lower chance of developing oligoanuria (<100 ml/m^2/day) than those who did not get diuretic medication [56].

In PD patients who need antihypertensive drugs and have RKF, the use of RAAS inhibitors, such as angiotensin converting enzyme (ACE) inhibitors or angiotensin II receptor blockers (ARB), should be taken into consideration. Kidney disease progression in children with ACE inhibitor use has been shown to be significantly slowed down [57]. Nevertheless, the IPPN also discovered that using RAAS inhibitors raised the likelihood of hyperkalemia considerably ($p = 0.04$) [54]. On the other hand, when an ACE inhibitor or an ARB is administered to PD patients, close monitoring for the existence of hyperkalemia is required. It is imperative that parents receive education regarding the temporary cessation of RAAS inhibitors for children who are at danger of dehydration, such as during a concurrent diarrheal sickness.

2.6 Solute clearance on PD

Our recommendation is to modify the PD prescription so as to bring the serum phosphate level back to normal. Children on PD should aim for a total minimum weekly Kt/V urea of 1.7, with adjustments made based on routine evaluations of clinical well-being and laboratory results, if necessary (*Level of evidence—Grade 2D)* [3].

Rationale: Because of the linked lower risk of cardiovascular disease and poorly controlled CKD-mineral bone disorder (MBD), improving phosphate removal and achieving a normal/near normal serum phosphorus level in children on PD is an important therapeutic aim.

A substantial correlation exists between abnormal bone micro-architecture and mineralization abnormalities and Ca status. Approximately 80% of children with CKD4-5 and 29% of those with CKD2 have mineralization defects [46]. In a similar vein, more than 90% of patients receiving peritoneal dialysis (PD) exhibited inadequate bone mineralization [58]. The length of time dialysate and peritoneal membrane are in touch determining how well phosphate is removed. Longer dwell times will therefore usually improve phosphate removal. The extended day stay should be optimized in individuals receiving APD and having an increased phosphate level. Peritoneal equilibration tests and the 24-hour dialytic phosphate clearance were evaluated in a study with 35 children on APD. The 2-hour dialysate/plasma phosphate ratio was a stronger predictor of the dialytic phosphate clearance than the creatinine equilibration features on the PET test. The dialytic phosphate clearance closely linked with the total dialysate turnover and the recommended number of cycles [59].

The mean blood phosphate level in the IPPN registry data was 1.8 + 0.5 mmol/l. It was negatively connected with the number of cycles, dwell time, and use of icodextrin, but directly correlated with the ultrafiltration volume [54]. Serum phosphate dropped by 0.17 mg/dl every hour dwell time and by 0.03 mg/dl per additional cycle, according to multivariate analysis [54]. Significantly, most dialysis patients require phosphate binders and dietary restrictions in order to reach normal phosphate levels; hence, the relative contributions of these factors, along with the effect of RKF on serum phosphate level, often influence the need for dialysis.

Regarding urea clearance, there are no conclusive studies in children that show a relationship between patient outcome or survival and dialytic or total (RKF and dialysis) Kt/Vurea. However, studies on HD in children that have demonstrated that, in contrast to traditional three times per week HD, faster growth rates are related to a higher Kt/V given through intensive dialysis regimens are of interest [60]. In its cohort of CPD patients, the IPPN registry has shown a mean dialytic Kt/Vurea of 2.24 + 0.84. Kt/Vurea was impacted by the APD prescription; daily ultrafiltration volume, number of cycles, and fill volumes during the day and night all had a significant direct impact on Kt/Vurea ($p < 0.001$).

Kt/Vurea rose by 0.02 for every 100 ml increase in ultrafiltration/day (adjusted for body surface area), with ultrafiltration volume showing the largest effect [54]. We propose that a total (dialysis and RKF) weekly Kt/Vurea of 1.7 be aimed in children, based on empirical data (poor) from the adult experience on a contribution of accomplished urea removal to patient outcome. To accomplish this aim, however, children with Kt/Vurea <1.7 who are otherwise responding well to PD should not have their prescription increased. This is based on a careful and frequent evaluation of clinical and laboratory indicators.

Patients on PD frequently have constipation, which can affect PD drainage and result in catheter migration. To prevent constipation, families need to be educated on the importance of keeping an eye on bowel motions and using laxatives—usually as a preventative measure.

2.7 Individualization of the prescription in PD

Optimizing fluid management and solute clearance is the aim of PD therapy, but it is important to take into account the child's and family's expectations regarding dialysis and quality of life. This will help the child make the most of their school and leisure time spent with friends and family [61]. For children with significant RKF, the dialysis program may need to be flexible, allowing for the occasional night without dialysis.

Similarly, if a child is on APD, it is best to restrict excessive fluid withdrawal, especially if the dialysate has a strong dextrose basis. This will reduce the possibility that the child will feel queasy and thirsty in the morning, which could negatively impact their performance or attendance at school. Without requiring frequent trips to the hospital, the use of remote monitoring equipment may enable appropriate monitoring of the child's health and modification of the PD prescription. A good long-term outcome may be attained by coordinating the aims of what the patient and doctor agree is "optimal" dialysis and negotiating an appropriate dialysis regimen with the patient and family ("shared decision-making").

Two groups of children were identified in the ESPN/ERA-EDTA Registry data based on when their dialysis was started: either <8 mL/min/1.73 m^2 (late starting) or ≥ 8 mL/min/1.73 m^2 (early initiation). They discovered that the groups' mean height SDS at the start of dialysis was 1.79 (95% CI 1.88 to 1.71) and 1.76 (95% CI 1.84 to 1.68) for early or late starters, respectively. The mean height SDS also demonstrated a malleable, significant, but comparable decline in the year following the start of dialysis (0.22 SDS for early and 0.24 SDS for late initiators) [16].

As part of high-quality care, the PD prescription should always be tailored to the specific medical and psychological needs of the patient and family. When evaluating the effectiveness of the dialysis regimen and the overall treatment regimen, equal consideration must be given to outcome parameters, such as growth, nutritional status, school attendance, and quality of life. While ultrafiltration, water and sodium balance, and solute purification are dialysis treatment targets that require appropriate modification of the fill volume, dwell time, and PD solution. Growth needs to be closely watched while taking into account dietary consumption, CKD-MBD management, acid-base status control, salt supplementation when necessary, and maybe recombinant growth hormone therapy. For the age-appropriate PD population, the use of nocturnal APD in dialysis regimens promotes school attendance. To find areas where changes to the overall treatment plan or more support may be needed, standardized assessments of health-related quality of life (HRQoL) should be carried out [26, 62]. Specifically, the "burden of care" related to the parents' and caregivers' provision of home PD needs to be continuously monitored, and the dialysis team should make support services accessible as needed [25].

2.8 Training

- We propose that PD training be conducted by a pediatric-trained, experienced PD nurse utilizing a structured teaching program with well-defined goals and standards that integrate adult learning concepts (2C).

- We propose that all caregivers receive periodic retraining. Additionally, we recommend that the PD approach be reevaluated following the onset of a peritonitis episode (2C).

2.8.1 Rationale

There are few systematic studies examining the training process itself and its relevance to patient outcomes, despite the fact that dialysis training is acknowledged to be critical to the effectiveness of PD programs and the avoidance of infections related to PD [63]. An international pediatric survey indicated that peritonitis rates were significantly lower ($p < 0.01$) in PD programs with longer training times and more patients, whereas recent international adult surveys found no correlation between training times and peritonitis rates [64].

In a previous recommendation, the ISPD stated that all new nephrology nurses should complete a minimum of 12 weeks of training and work in a PD unit. This should include 6–8 weeks of orientation under the guidance of an experienced PD nurse, during which time they should observe procedures, educate patients, and provide clinical care [65]. The ISPD has suggested, more recently, that before new PD trainers can work as independent trainers, they should be monitored for at least one patient training course [63]. The pediatric workgroup concurs with the ISPD Nursing Liaison Committee that, in order for a PD training program to be considered effective, the student must be able to satisfy (at the very least) these three objectives, even though the ideal length of training is yet unknown.

- Carry out all necessary operations safely.
- Identify contamination and infection.
- Enumerate every suitable reaction to contamination and infection.

To avoid infection and contamination, wash your hands frequently. Before beginning any care operation, caregivers must be instructed to wash their hands thoroughly [66]. After hand washing, it is crucial to thoroughly dry your hands with a clean towel to prevent bacterial translocation by contact contamination [67]. It is standard procedure and advised in pediatric programs to train two family members or caregivers, one of whom may be the patient if judged capable [68].

2.9 Conclusion

Through strict adherence to PD catheter care packages, quality improvement initiatives such as the Standardizing Care to Improve Outcomes in Pediatric ESRD effort have effectively shown a decrease in peritonitis rates [69]. Improvement science techniques like these have aided in determining the main variables that are directly related to the outcome of peritonitis and the part that variables such as patient and family engagement tactics and health literacy may play in enhancing the prognosis of children with PD [70].

All newborns, children, and teenagers receiving chronic PD should have their nondialysis care managed in compliance with the pediatric-specific information found in the following guidelines: the KDIGO Guidelines for the Management of Anemia in Chronic Kidney Disease (CKD) [50], the KDIGO Clinical Practice Guidelines for the Management of Blood Pressure in CKD [49], the KDIGO Guidelines for Lipid Management in CKD [71], the KDOQI Clinical Practice Guidelines for Nutrition in Children with CKD [22], and the guidelines from the European Society of Pediatric Nephrology for the management of CKD-MBD [72, 73].

Given that ESKD affects several organ systems, clinical therapy of a juvenile patient with chronic PD necessitates attention to a wide range of clinical concerns that may be present. Optimizing care is the goal of incorporating the many published suggestions into clinical care. It is acknowledged that most recommendations are supported by both expert opinion and evidence.

3. Acute peritoneal dialysis

3.1 Introduction

Acute kidney injury (AKI) is a frequent side effect among ill children in hospitals. AKI prevalence varies from 5 to 25% in both non-critical and critical patients according to research employing current classifications. In all age categories, there is an independent correlation between it and higher rates of morbidity and mortality [74–77]. The mortality rate for these youngsters is significantly higher in areas where dialysis is needed but not readily available [78]. The first renal replacement therapy (RRT) modality utilized to treat AKI in children of all ages was PD. In certain regions of the world, its use has decreased in favor of the more recent extracorporeal blood purification technology. According to a recent internet survey, the most popular dialysis modalities for AKI in children in high-income countries (HIC), primarily in North America, were continuous renal replacement therapy (CRRT) at 24% and hemodialysate (HD) at 72% in HIC countries, while 68% of infants in low- and lower middle-income countries (LLMIC) were dialyzed with PD [79]. On the other hand, intermittent HD (22.4%), PD, and CRRT (39.4 and 38.2%, respectively) were the most commonly reported dialysis modalities, according to a recent survey conducted across 35 pediatric nephrology centers in Europe.

PD was the most frequently selected modality in centers treating patients following heart surgery [80]. The patient's clinical qualities and the socioeconomic and geographic context appear to have an impact on the treatment mode selection. The application of extracorporeal techniques in children is still costly, complex, and dependent on technology, and requires experienced specialized nursing personnel. This makes it challenging to implement in areas with limited resources, even with advancements in technology and the development of safety procedures.

With new devices (PD cyclers) that have improved safety profiles, fewer connections, and the ability to provide a wider range of PD prescriptions, PD has also benefited from technical advancements. Nonetheless, in LLMIC, manual methods are still more frequently employed. PD can be carried out manually with closed manual exchange systems in premature and small newborns for whom APD cycler systems are unable to supply small enough amounts. These low-cost manual exchange devices can be used with even the tiniest newborns, such as those with severe and very low birthweights [81–83]. Nephrotoxic medications, cardiopulmonary bypass, and low cardiac output can all result in fluid overload (FO), which puts children and newborns having heart surgery at high risk for AKI.

Conversely, PD catheters are frequently inserted during difficult cardiac surgery in numerous pediatric cardiac centers in highly resourced nations, particularly in the youngest newborns. As part of post-operative treatment, early PD (on the day of surgery or post-operative day 1) has been started utilizing either PD or passive drainage *via* the PD catheter. Research on the effects of these procedures have revealed reduced electrolyte imbalances, shorter times on mechanical breathing, and earlier times for negative fluid balance [84].

Despite the fact that PD is commonly used in the treatment of AKI, no RCTs have been conducted to compare the efficacy or results of various renal replacement modalities for the treatment of AKI in children, in contrast to the adult literature [85]. Clinical practice guidelines for the use of PD in the treatment of AKI in children are presented by the ISPD in order to improve survival in children [86].

4. Peritoneal dialysis practice in children

Under the direction of the ISPD, these recommendations were created. The GRADE system, a thoroughly tested framework that balances recommendation strength and evidence level, serves as the foundation for the recommendations [87]. A recommendation of grade 1 is strongly advised, but one of grade 2 is not. The suggestions' level of evidence is indicated by the letters (A through D). A practice point was designated for situations in which there is insufficient evidence to support a committee's suggestion, but there is sufficient clinical experience to do so.

Since they are guidelines, practice patterns should be guided by them. It is crucial to remember, nevertheless, that not all clinical circumstances will fall under the recommendations' purview. Instead, clinicians should use the knowledge at their disposal to provide patients with the best treatment possible, acknowledging that there may be times when deviating from the guidelines is required.

4.1 Peritoneal dialysis is a suitable renal replacement therapy modality for the treatment of AKI in children (1C)

4.1.1 Rationale

4.1.1.1 Implementation simplicity

Because it is less expensive and requires less technical expertise than both continuous extracorporeal treatments and HD, PD is especially helpful in areas with limited infrastructure [88–90]. Studies conducted in the past have demonstrated that children with hemodynamic instability and multi-organ failure needing vasopressors can safely undergo PD [91, 92]. With the use of bedside dialysis catheters, therapy can be started quickly, safely, and without the requirement for anticoagulation. Additionally, for patients whose conditions are stable, this may remove the requirement for an intensive care unit (ICU). Although severe fluid restriction in infants increases the risk of hypoglycemia, the use of glucose-containing PD solutions and the treated patients' subsequent absorption of glucose allow for severe fluid restriction in infants with AKI without increasing that risk.

4.1.1.2 Alternative with other therapies

There is no difference in mortality between children treated with PD and those getting CRRT as treatment for AKI, according to observational studies comparing modalities. A 1995 retrospective analysis by Fleming et al. on 34 children who had heart surgery revealed that, in comparison with PD, CRRT was linked to improved nutritional support and fluid control [93]. On the other hand, mortality did not vary. In 2001 [92], retrospective examination of 226 children with AKI from different sources revealed no difference in mortality between PD and CRRT. In every disease condition examined in this investigation, HD outlived CRRT or PD in terms of survival. The authors explained the higher HD survival rate by pointing out that a higher number of hemodynamically stable HD patients were preselected for the disease.

In 136 children, ages 1 month to 16 years, a retrospective study from India compared the safety and effectiveness of continuous PD vs. daily intermittent HD. It indicated that children receiving HD had a 75% higher risk of dying than those receiving PD [94]. The HD children in this study experienced recurrent hypotensive episodes while receiving medication, and fluid and electrolyte imbalances were identified as potential causes of death in a risk analysis. Krause et al. conducted a retrospective investigation of 115 children in Israel who were undergoing dialysis for AKI. The results showed that intermittent HD was linked with a considerably better outcome than either hemodiafiltration (HDF) or PD [95]. The authors mentioned that patients on PD and HDF received stronger vasopressor support as potential explanations for this result.

The fact that the patients on PD and HDF were younger and that the PD group was considerably bigger than the other groups could potentially have had an impact on the result. The small number of patients, the lack of standardization in the therapy given, the variability in the modalities available, and the additional variability in the modalities' expertise and experience all hindered these studies, as they do many pediatric investigations. The varying results are most likely explained by these factors. One issue that many LLMIC face is that HD in adult units is frequently the only readily available dialysis modality for children. As a result, excessively quick clearances and significant intravascular volume shifts are caused by non-pediatric circuits and filters. PD would be helpful in these circumstances.

In summary, there is currently no definite advantage of one dialysis technique over another for the management of AKI. PD is an effective therapy option for AKI in young people of all shapes and sizes.

4.1.2 Selection of the modality

Since there is currently no evidence to support any particular modality over another, as was previously discussed, the choice of modality in areas where all RRT modalities are accessible typically comes down to personal preference and local expertise. That being said, PD might be preferred over other modalities in the following circumstances:

a. Due to the challenge of inserting vascular catheters big enough to permit extracorporeal methods, PD is often the dialysis option used in low birthweight neonates [81–83].

b. Small newborns following heart surgery [84, 96].

c. The existence of bleeding diatheses that make big central venous catheter implantation contraindicated.

d. Cardiovascular instability in infants too tiny for low extracorporeal blood volume because specialist pediatric CRRT equipment is not easily accessible. The advantages of acute PD are seen in **Table 2**.

4.2 Fluid supply and access for pediatric acute PD

- The best option for PD access is a Tenckhoff catheter that is implanted by a surgeon in the operating room. (1B) (optimal).

- Using an insertion kit and the Seldinger procedure to introduce a PD catheter is a suitable substitute. (1C) (optimal)

- An acceptable substitute is the interventional radiological implantation of PD catheters using a combination of fluoroscopy and ultrasound. (1D) (optimal)
- To reduce the risk of problems, rigid catheters inserted with a stylet should only be used in the absence of soft Seldinger catheters and for no more than 3 days. (1C) (minimum standard).
- When a normal PD access is unavailable, improvised PD catheters should only be utilized. (Practice point)(Minimum standard).
- Before inserting a PD catheter, we advise using prophylactic antibiotics. (1B) (optimal)
- It is recommended to utilize a closed delivery system with a Y connection. (1A) (optimal). When doing manual physical therapy on young children, a system that uses buretrols to measure fill and drainage volumes should be employed. (Practice point)(Optimal).
- In environments with limited resources, an open system with bag spiking may be employed; however, this system should be planned to minimize the quantity of possible contamination sites and guarantee accurate fill and drainage volume measurements. (Practice point) (Minimum standard).
- Automated peritoneal dialysis is appropriate for treating pediatric AKI, with the exception of newborns whose fill volumes are too tiny for the machines that are currently on the market. (1D).

4.2.1 Rationale

4.2.1.1 Catheter types and insertion

Surgical (open dissection or laparoscopic), blind percutaneous utilizing a Seldinger approach, interventional radiological placement, and rigid catheters put

Advantages of acute PD
Simplicity
Minimal infrastructural support
Irrespective to disruption of power and limited accessibility to clean water
Less financial cost than HD or CRRT especially in developing countries
Avoidance of vascular access in infants
Possibility in small newborns following heart surgery
Indication in case of hemodynamic instability
No need for anticoagulation
Continuous ultrafiltration
Nutritional support

Table 2.
Advantages of acute PD in children and infants.

with a stylet are among the catheter implantation techniques utilized for acute PD. Catheter insertion techniques are typically determined by the patient's needs and the expertise that are accessible locally.

4.2.1.2 Catheters inserted surgically

For pediatric patients with acute PD, the best option is an operating room Tenckhoff catheter placed by a surgeon [91, 97–99]. This has worked well even with young infants. It has been demonstrated that laparoscopic Tenckhoff PD catheter insertion in children is equally successful as open surgical operations, with no discernible variations in the rates of complications [100]. It is also helpful to perform laparoscopic salvage of migrating or obstructed catheters [101]. Because port site suturing minimizes leakage, laparoscopy may be preferable to laparotomy in this case. During the procedure, the heart surgeons in numerous locations will implant a Tenckhoff catheter. These catheters can be implanted using a variety of procedures [102]. This placement of the catheters typically results in a low rate of complications [96, 103, 104]. There is a higher likelihood of a rupture between the peritoneum and the pleural space in children who have had sternotomies. This problem may or may not develop depending on the particular procedure the heart surgeon used to implant the catheter.

4.2.1.3 Catheters placed by Seldinger technique

An appropriate substitute for surgical catheter implantation in children of all sizes is bedside catheter insertion utilizing the Seldinger technique with soft, flexible Cook or Tenckhoff catheters. Either the Cook Mac-LocTM Multi-purpose Drainage Catheters (CMMDC) or the temporary Cook PD catheters, which have been used successfully for many years [92, 93, 105, 106], are the Cook catheters that are employed. A mean age of 6.9 months was seen in 21 infants and toddlers who received these multifunctional catheters. Only three of the patients' problems prevented PD from continuing. The catheter was used by the remaining patients until either non-renal death or recovery from AKI. There were no infections linked to the catheter and good target fluid and solute clearance were attained. At day 14, 90% of the catheters survived, with a mean of 10.5 (range 2–29) days without complications.

4.2.1.4 Interventional radiological placement

Compared to standard surgical placement, interventional radiological placement of PD catheters using fluoroscopy and ultrasound in adults is a less intrusive, safer, more affordable, and equally effective approach. Adult consensus protocols are available, which enables urgent-start PD for patients who arrive late at ESKF and require dialysis. Additionally, it permits a single process that might be adequate for both acute and ongoing dialysis accesses. Although there is no information about this method in children, its use may be able to prevent the requirement for transient vascular access catheters by employing vessels that can be challenging to access and may become damaged with long-term consequences. Fluoroscopy machines may be scarce in less developed nations, while ultrasound machines are becoming more widely available in pediatric hospitals across the globe.

4.2.1.5 Rigid stylet insertion PD catheters

Rigid stylet PD catheters can be utilized in lieu of soft Seldinger-inserted catheters. It is not recommended to use rigid stylet catheters for longer than 2 to 3 days because of the increased risk of leakage, dislodgement, viscus damage, and peritonitis [99, 107]. Nonetheless, these catheters are usually easily accessible and reasonably priced. According to a Sudanese study, PD was the most often used dialysis modality for 659 children with AKI over a 7-year period (343 children, or 52.4%). A blind procedure was successfully used to put a rigid catheter (Peritocat, peritoneal dialysis catheter, B. Braun Melsungen AG, Melsunge, Germany) at the patient's bedside. PD was administered for an average of 4.5 days (range: 2–9 days).

A soft PD catheter was implanted or the patient was converted to HD when dialysis was required for an extended length of time. In addition to bowel, bladder, and vascular damage in 7 cases, 53 patients (15.4%) also had peritonitis as a result of the hard stylet. On the other hand, 450 children (68.9%) recovered from AKI overall, and 205/343 (65.4%) recovered following PD [108].

4.2.2 Manual PD delivery systems

For newborns and children with AKI, PD may be administered manually using a gravity-based device. Closed systems are linked to lower rates of peritonitis when compared to normal spiking systems [109, 110]. Buretrols help with strict fluid balance, which is crucial for the very young and allows for accurate assessment of intake and drainage. Additionally, by reducing the number of connections, this strategy lowers the chance of contact contamination. The PD-Paed system (Fresenius Medical Care, Bad Homburg, Germany), the Baxter manual PD system, and the Dialy-Nate system/Gesco Dialy-nate (Utah Medical Products, Midvale, Utah, USA) planned for commercial release are among the systems now in use.

4.2.3 Automated PD systems

APD provides a large range of extremely effective treatment plans that are derived from individualized intraperitoneal volumes (IPVs), high dialysate flow rates, and brief dwell durations. APD has the benefit of not requiring as much intensive nursing care, but it is more expensive.

4.3 Dialysis solutions for acute PD in children

- Dextrose should be added to the acute peritoneal dialysis solution at a concentration that will allow for the desired level of ultrafiltration. (Practice Point)

- Potassium should be introduced to dialysate sterilely as soon as serum potassium levels drop to less than 4 mmol/l. (Practice Point) (optimal) After 12 hours of continuous PD, potassium should be empirically added to the dialysis solution to reach a dialysate concentration of 3–5 mmol/l if facilities for measuring serum potassium are lacking. (Practice point) (Minimum standard)

- After serum electrolyte concentrations stabilize, measurements should be made every day after the initial 24 hours. (Practice Point)(optimal) When resources are scarce, daily measurements of potassium and sodium should be made (practice point) (minimum standard).

- It is best to utilize solutions containing bicarbonate when there is hepatic dysfunction, hemodynamic instability, and persistent or worsening metabolic acidosis. (>1D) (Optimal) An alternative is to employ lactate-containing solutions in situations where these solutions are unavailable. (2D) (minimum standard)

- It is recommended to utilize commercially prepared dialysis solutions. (1C) (Optimal) Locally prepared fluids, however, may be used in situations when resources do not allow for them, provided that sterile preparation protocols and patient outcomes—such as the incidence of peritonitis—are closely monitored (1C) (minimal standard).

4.3.1 Rationale

4.3.1.1 Acute PD fluids' dextrose contents

Acute PD solutions with dextrose concentrations of 1.5, 2.5, and 4.25% are typically sold commercially (if glucose is measured, the comparable concentrations are 1.36, 2.27, or 3.86%). The 1.5, 2.5, and 4.25% solutions have osmolality values of 346, 396, and 485 mosmol/l, respectively. When these solutions are used, an osmotic gradient is created between the dialysate and plasma, which facilitates the evacuation of fluid [111]. Small exchange volumes, which are usually employed for acute PD, facilitate glucose absorption across the peritoneal membrane continuously and progressively reduce the osmolar gradient and reduce the efficiency of ultrafiltration. Conversely, when FO is present, acute PD is typically started with a 2.5% dextrose solution to facilitate efficient ultrafiltration, and a minimal fill volume is advised to prevent dialysate leakage.

In cases of euvolemia or mild FO, a 1.5% solution may be used initially. Particularly in young infants, using a 2.5% or 4.25% solution in a PD prescription with frequent exchanges might cause hyperglycemia, which may require insulin therapy or a reduction in the amount of dextrose used.

4.3.2 Serum electrolytes and dialysate

At the start of treatment, the potassium concentration in the dialysis solution should be very low (1–2 mmol/l), since many patients will have hyperkalemia, which is frequently accompanied by metabolic acidosis. The concentration of potassium in the dialysis solution can be gradually increased to a concentration of 4 mmol/l once a normal serum potassium concentration is reached, which usually happens during the first 6–12 hours of dialysis. Further adjustments will depend on factors that affect the serum potassium level, such as the concentration of dialysate dextrose, serum CO_2, medications, parenteral nutrition. Consideration should be made to the empirical addition of potassium to the dialysis solution after 12 hours of continuous PD in order to reach a dialysate concentration of 3–5 mmol/l if there are no facilities to monitor serum potassium. Potassium losses in acute PD can be substantial, and potassium depletion and cardiovascular instability might result from its removal. One possible way to avoid or treat hypokalemia is to incorporate potassium (4 mmol/l) into the dialysis solution [112, 113].

In order to avoid precipitation, supplemental calcium must be administered by a different method than in the PD solution. When the dialysate has a high bicarbonate concentration, it is necessary to constantly monitor serum ionized calcium levels in order to support measures intended to stop tetany from developing. It should be mentioned that convective clearance causes bicarbonate loss from dialysate to increase in correlation with high ultrafiltration rates [114]. About 132–134 mmol/l is the normal concentration of sodium in dialysate. Since there is not much of a concentration difference between dialysate and plasma, convection is mostly used for sodium transfer.

Most free water is removed in the first 30 to 60 minutes of each exchange. Lowering the concentration of glucose in the dialysis solution or, if solute clearance permits, lengthening the dwell duration should be taken into account if hypernatremia occurs. In order to match the net ultrafiltration from PD, a hypotonic fluid, such as 0.45% saline, can be administered intravenously if rapid cycling is required for solute removal and fluid balance is neutral or negative.

4.3.3 PD fluids based on bicarbonate

Alkali in the dialysate aids in reversing any acidosis that may accompany AKI. While lactate-based dialysis solutions, which are commonly available in the United States, are commonly used for acute APD in children, more biocompatible solutions, such as bicarbonate or lactate/bicarbonate-based solutions, are available in other countries [115]. Occasionally, when there are persistent or worsening metabolic acidosis, hemodynamic instability, and hepatic dysfunction, newborns and young children cannot handle the lactate absorbed from the dialysis solution. It is best to use a bicarbonate-based solution that has been made commercially or by a pharmacist in these circumstances.

Although there are no data specifically on children in this area, there is not much evidence in the adult literature to support a bicarbonate solution's superiority over a lactate-based solution in terms of clinically significant outcomes such as adverse events and death. But in the single adult randomized controlled trial, patients in shock treated with bicarbonate-based PD fluids had a markedly improved pH, bicarbonate level, and lactate level when compared to patients treated with lactate-based solutions [116].

4.4 Acute PD prescriptions for pediatric patients

- To reduce the possibility of dialysate leakage, the first fill volume should be kept to 10–20 ml/kg. If the patient is able to tolerate it, the volume can then be gradually increased to about 30–40 ml/kg (800–1100 ml/m^2). (Practice Point)

- The first exchange duration, which includes the inflow, dwell, and drain times, should normally take place every 60 to 90 minutes. As fluid and solute removal targets are met, a gradual extension of the dwell time can take place. It could be necessary to shorten the cycle time in newborns and early babies in order to achieve sufficient ultrafiltration. (Practice Point)

- To establish and maintain normotension and euvolemia, close monitoring of total fluid intake and outflow is required. (1B)

- throughout the first 3 days of therapy, acute PD should be sustained throughout the entire twenty-four-hour period. (1C)

- When giving acute PD, careful monitoring of medication dosages and levels should be done, if available. (Practice Point)

4.4.1 Fill volumes

When starting acute PD and shortly after PD catheter implantation, small fill volumes are typically advised to reduce the possibility of dialysate leakage due to the intraperitoneal pressure (IPP) rise generated by the PD solution [85].

Since bigger volumes result in longer prolonged maintenance of the concentration and osmolar gradients, the fill volume can be gradually raised to maximize solute and fluid evacuation if no leakage occurs [117].

For patients younger than 2 years old, the fill volume should generally not be more than 800 ml/m^2 due to the possibility of an increase in IPP and the subsequent lymphatic reabsorption of full traffic [51].

Fill volumes greater than 40 ml/kg (1100 ml/m^2) are infrequently necessary if PD is prescribed on a continuous schedule, and they may affect breathing in an ICU [118].

4.4.2 Duration of exchange

In order to achieve the intended ultrafiltration and solute removal while maintaining the gradients between serum and dialysate, short exchange periods are first employed. Even so, exchange times as short as 60 minutes have been employed occasionally. One such instance is detailed in a recent literature review on postpartum depression in extremely low birthweight (<1000 g) and very low birthweight (<1500 g) premature babies, wherein shorter dwell times (10–20 min) and smaller fill volumes (7–14 ml) were effectively employed [82].

Since filling and draining a patient takes a significant amount of time, solute clearance is frequently hampered [119].

4.4.3 Fluid volume

AKI in pediatric patients is often coupled with hypervolemia, and a significant FO has been linked to a higher risk of morbidity and death [120]. For many patients, the elimination of fluid is a major therapy goal, and fluid balance must be constantly monitored. The capacity to reach a specified fluid goal should, in most situations, be reevaluated at least every 2–3 hours at first, and therapy should then be modified as needed.

The ideal situation would be one in which the patient's fluid needs for medication, blood products, nutrition, and hemodynamic stability are met while simultaneously resolving the fluid overloaded state due to the successful generation of ultrafiltrate with each exchange (plus any urine output that may exist). Hypertonic dialysis solutions (2.5/4.25%) and frequent exchanges early in the course of acute PD when the fill volumes are small are often necessary to regularly achieve positive ultrafiltration and meet the patient's needs; modification of the ultrafiltration needs will mandate the adjustment of the dialysis prescription.

4.4.4 PD time

To address the patient's needs for solute and fluid removal during the first phase of stabilization, acute PD should typically be used continuously with frequent exchanges. The patient's clinical situation should dictate how frequently exchanges occur. The effectiveness of PD for treating AKI is sometimes limited by the modest fill volume that commonly defines the initial prescription; as a result, PD usually needs to be sustained for the entire 24-hour period in the acute setting in order to obtain appropriate clearances and fluid evacuation. There is currently no information linking clearances to results in kids with acute PD. Consequently, it is impossible to determine a target dialysis dose; 75 l/week/1.73 m^2 was the weekly average creatinine clearance in two pediatric trials of AKI induced by a wide range of etiologies when a fill volume of 20 ml/kg and a well time of 60 min were employed [121, 122].

4.4.5 Modification of medication dosage

As a patient moves from AKI with oliguria to PD, numerous medications may no longer be cleared. This could lead to insufficient serum levels, particularly when using medications such as antibiotics and anticonvulsants, therefore dosage needs to be changed appropriately.

5. Handling PD-related issues for AKI

The use of PD to treat AKI in children is related to several possible risks. The following will be briefly mentioned, even though a detailed examination of them is outside the purview of these guidelines:

- peritonitis,
- mechanical issues,
- protein loss, and
- hyperglycemia.

5.1 Peritonitis

Major consequence of acute PD is peritonitis. The rates of infection varied significantly between centers [123–125]. These instructions include recommendations to lower the rate of infection that are unique to acute PD. It should be noted that the patient's overall sickness may hide the clinical indications of peritonitis, and that the patient's overall inflammatory condition may affect the patient's likelihood of fulfilling the diagnostic criteria for chronic PD peritonitis. Therefore, it seems sense to think about monitoring for peritonitis in individuals receiving acute PD by doing a leukocyte count every day.

5.2 Mechanical issues with catheters inserted using a Seldinger technique (cook)

Ten to fifty percent of Seldinger catheter placement cases result in access dysfunction [92, 98, 126]. Access dysfunction has been observed to occur far less frequently when the soft coiled multipurpose catheters are used [127, 128]. Catheter blockage and peri-catheter leaking are the most often reported access-related problems.

5.3 Mechanical issues with Tenckhoff catheters that are tunneled

Three to thirty percent of children who have a tunneled Tenckhoff PD catheter may experience access problems [92, 97, 129]. The treatment of children's tunneled

Tenckhoff catheter access dysfunction is identical to that of adults. (For more on PD in AKI and ISPD criteria for establishing and preserving ideal PD access, see the adult ISPD guidelines [130, 131]).

5.4 Protein loss in PD

Acute PD can cause protein loss from the peritoneal membrane, which can impair the patient's immune system and nutrition [132, 133]. Throughout treatment, it is imperative that patients receive enough nutrition, particularly additional protein supplements, ideally with the assistance of a nutritionist. Patients should generally be given the amount of protein lost during dialysis in addition to the dietary reference intakes. The KDOQI pediatric nutrition guidelines take into account the average daily quantities lost due to chronic PD [22].

5.5 Hyperglycemia

In acute PD, there is a risk of developing hyperglycemia because of the high glucose concentration in PD fluid. In order to facilitate the best possible ultrafiltration, this should be treated since it lowers the osmotic gradient between serum and PD fluid. It has also been demonstrated that maintaining normoglycemia considerably increases critically sick patients' chances of survival.

6. Conclusion

Dialysis for AKI is still a challenging procedure that needs experience. The studies show significant advancements in the use of peritoneal dialysis as a pediatric renal replacement therapy in AKI, along with ongoing difficulties. The technique's survival rate has significantly increased over the last 20 years, but infectious and mechanical complications reduce the method's viability. The International Society for Peritoneal Dialysis extensively review the available literature and present updated recommendations for PD in AKI in pediatrics regarding peritoneal access, dialysis solutions, treatment of fluid control, and prescription of dialysis. Finally, these guidelines are designed to improve the outcome of children who receive PD.

Author details

Souad Chelghoum*, Salah-eddine Benfarhi and Atmane Seba
Nephrology Department, Nefissa Hamoud Hospital, Hussein-Dey University Hospital Center, Algiers, Algeria

*Address all correspondence to: souadchelghoum399@gmail.com

References

[1] Rees L, Schaefer F, Schmitt CP, Shroff R, Warady BA. Chronic dialysis in children and adolescents: Challenges and outcomes. The Lancet Child & Adolescent Health. 2017;**1**(1):68-77

[2] Warady BA, Schaefer F, Bagga A, Cano F, McCulloch M, Yap HK, et al. Prescribing peritoneal dialysis for high-quality care in children. Peritoneal Dialysis International: Journal of the International Society for Peritoneal Dialysis. 2020;**40**(3):333-340

[3] Brown EA, Blake PG, Boudville N, Davies S, De Arteaga J, Dong J, et al. International Society for Peritoneal Dialysis practice recommendations: Prescribing high-quality goal-directed peritoneal dialysis. Peritoneal Dialysis International: Journal of the International Society for Peritoneal Dialysis. 2020;**40**(3):244-253

[4] Teitelbaum I, Glickman J, Neu A, Neumann J, Rivara MB, Shen J, et al. KDOQI US commentary on the 2020 ISPD practice recommendations for prescribing high-quality goal-directed peritoneal dialysis. American Journal of Kidney Diseases. 2021;**77**(2):157-171

[5] Corbett RW, Goodlet G, MacLaren B, Jolliffe A, Joseph A, Lu C, et al. International Society for Peritoneal Dialysis Practice Recommendations: The view of the person who is doing or who has done peritoneal dialysis. Peritoneal Dialysis International: Journal of the International Society for Peritoneal Dialysis. 2020;**40**(3):349-352

[6] Karava V, Stabouli S, Dotis J, Liakopoulos V, Papachristou F, Printza N. Tracking hydration status changes by bioimpedance spectroscopy in children on peritoneal dialysis. Peritoneal Dialysis International: Journal of the International Society for Peritoneal Dialysis. 2021;**41**(2):217-225

[7] Dasgupta I, Keane D, Lindley E, Shaheen I, Tyerman K, Schaefer F, et al. Validating the use of bioimpedance spectroscopy for assessment of fluid status in children. Pediatric Nephrology. 2018;**33**(9):1601-1607

[8] Eng CSY, Bhowruth D, Mayes M, Stronach L, Blaauw M, Barber A, et al. Assessing the hydration status of children with chronic kidney disease and on dialysis: A comparison of techniques. Nephrology, Dialysis, Transplantation. 2018;**33**(5):847-855

[9] Oh KH, Baek SH, Joo KW, Kim DK, Kim YS, Kim S, et al. Does routine bioimpedance-guided fluid management provide additional benefit to non-Anuric peritoneal dialysis patients? Results from compass clinical trial. Peritoneal Dialysis International: Journal of the International Society for Peritoneal Dialysis. 2018;**38**(2):131-138

[10] Yoon HE, Kwon YJ, Shin SJ, Lee S, Lee S, Kim S, et al. Bioimpedance spectroscopy-guided fluid management in peritoneal dialysis patients with residual kidney function: A randomized controlled trial. Nephrology. 2019;**24**(12):1279-1289

[11] Hennessy K, Capparelli EV, Romanowski G, Alejandro L, Murray W, Benador N. Intraperitoneal vancomycin for peritoneal dialysis-associated peritonitis in children: Evaluation of loading dose guidelines. Peritoneal Dialysis International: Journal of the International Society for Peritoneal Dialysis. 2021;**41**(2):202-208

[12] Warady BA, Bakkaloglu S, Newland J, Cantwell M, Verrina E, Neu A, et al. Consensus Guidelines for the prevention and treatment of catheter-related infections and peritonitis in Pediatric patients receiving peritoneal dialysis: 2012 update. Peritoneal Dialysis International: Journal of the International Society for Peritoneal Dialysis. 2012;**32**(Suppl. 2):32-86

[13] Borzych-Dużałka D, Schaefer F, Warady BA. Targeting optimal PD management in children: What have we learned from the IPPN registry? Pediatric Nephrology. 2021;**36**(5):1053-1063

[14] Neu AM, Richardson T, Lawlor J, Stuart J, Newland J, McAfee N, et al. Implementation of standardized follow-up care significantly reduces peritonitis in children on chronic peritoneal dialysis. Kidney International. 2016;**89**(6):1346-1354

[15] Winnicki E, Johansen KL, Cabana MD, Warady BA, McCulloch CE, Grimes B, et al. Higher eGFR at dialysis initiation is not associated with a survival benefit in children. Journal of the American Society of Nephrology : JASN. 2019;**30**(8):1505-1513

[16] Preka E, Bonthuis M, Harambat J, Jager KJ, Groothoff JW, Baiko S, et al. Association between timing of dialysis initiation and clinical outcomes in the paediatric population: An ESPN/ERA-EDTA registry study. Nephrology, Dialysis, Transplantation. 2019;**34**(11):1932-1940

[17] Preka E, Rees L. Should we abandon GFR in the decision to initiate chronic dialysis? Pediatric Nephrology. 2020;**35**(9):1593-1600

[18] Schwartz GJ, Muñoz A, Schneider MF, Mak RH, Kaskel F, Warady BA, et al. New equations to estimate GFR in children with CKD. Journal of the American Society of Nephrology : JASN. 2009;**20**(3):629-637

[19] Salvador CL, Tøndel C, Rowe AD, Bjerre A, Brun A, Brackman D, et al. Estimating glomerular filtration rate in children: Evaluation of creatinine- and cystatin C-based equations. Pediatric Nephrology. 2019;**34**(2):301-311

[20] Weaver DJ, Somers MJG, Martz K, Mitsnefes MM. Clinical outcomes and survival in pediatric patients initiating chronic dialysis: A report of the NAPRTCS registry. Pediatric Nephrology. 2017;**32**(12):2319-2330

[21] USRDS. Annual Report. CKD among children and adolescents. Chapter 6. 2018

[22] National Kidney Foundation. KDOQI clinical practice guideline for nutrition in children with CKD: 2008 update. American Journal of Kidney Diseases. 2009;**53**(3):S11-S104

[23] Jain AK, Blake P, Cordy P, Garg AX. Global trends in rates of peritoneal dialysis. Journal of the American Society of Nephrology : JASN. 2012;**23**(3):533-544

[24] Fischbach M, Zaloszyc A, Schaefer B, Schmitt CP. Optimizing peritoneal dialysis prescription for volume control: The importance of varying dwell time and dwell volume. Pediatric Nephrology. 2014;**29**(8):1321-1327

[25] Watson AR. Stress and burden of care in families with children commencing renal replacement therapy. Advances in Peritoneal Dialysis. Conference on Peritoneal Dialysis. 1997;**13**:300-304

[26] Goldstein SL, Graham N, Warady BA, Seikaly M, McDonald R,

Burwinkle TM, et al. Measuring health-related quality of life in children with ESRD: Performance of the generic and ESRD-specific instrument of the Pediatric quality of life inventory (PedsQL). American Journal of Kidney Diseases. 2008;**51**(2):285-297

[27] Chadha V, Blowey DL, Warady BA. Is growth a valid outcome measure of dialysis clearance in children undergoing peritoneal dialysis? Peritoneal Dialysis International: Journal of the International Society for Peritoneal Dialysis. 2001;**21**(Suppl. 3):S179-S184

[28] Termorshuizen F, Dekker FW, Van Manen JG, Korevaar JC, Boeschoten EW, Krediet RT. Relative contribution of residual renal function and different measures of adequacy to survival in Hemodialysis patients: An analysis of the Netherlands cooperative study on the adequacy of dialysis (NECOSAD)-2. Journal of the American Society of Nephrology : JASN. 2004;**15**(4):1061-1070

[29] Bargman JM, Thorpe KE, Churchill DN. Relative contribution of residual renal function and peritoneal clearance to adequacy of dialysis: A reanalysis of the CANUSA study. Journal of the American Society of Nephrology : JASN. 2001;**12**(10):2158-2162

[30] Misra M, Vonesh E, Van Stone JC, Moore HL, Prowant B, Nolph KD. Effect of cause and time of dropout on the residual GFR: A comparative analysis of the decline of GFR on dialysis. Kidney International. 2001;**59**(2):754-763

[31] Feber J, Scharer K, Schaefer F, Mikova M, Janda J. Residual renal function in children on haemodialysis and peritoneal dialysis therapy. Pediatric Nephrology. 1994;**8**(5):579-583

[32] Maya ID. Ambulatory setting for peritoneal dialysis catheter placement. Seminars in Dialysis. 2008;**21**(5):457-458

[33] Maya ID. Ultrasound/fluoroscopy-assisted placement of peritoneal dialysis catheters. Seminars in Dialysis. 2007;**20**(6):611-615

[34] Zaman F, Pervez A, Atray NK, Murphy S, Work J, Abreo KD. Fluoroscopy-assisted placement of peritoneal dialysis catheters by nephrologists. Seminars in Dialysis. 2005;**18**(3):247-251

[35] Asif A. American Society of Diagnostic and Interventional Nephrology Section Editor: Stephen Ash: Peritoneal dialysis access-related procedures by nephrologists. Seminars in Dialysis. 2004;**17**(5):398-406

[36] Crabtree JH. Is the Tenckhoff catheter still the first choice for use with peritoneal dialysis? Seminars in Dialysis. 2011;**24**(4):447-448

[37] Ash SR, Bever SL. Peritoneal dialysis for acute renal failure: The safe, effective, and low-cost modality. Advances in Renal Replacement Therapy. 1995;**2**(2):160-163

[38] Burdmann EA, Chakravarthi R. Peritoneal dialysis in acute kidney injury: Lessons learned and applied. Seminars in Dialysis. 2011;**24**(2):149-156

[39] Guidelines Committee SAGES, Haggerty S, Roth S, Walsh D, Stefanidis D, Price R, et al. Guidelines for laparoscopic peritoneal dialysis access surgery. Surgical Endoscopy. 2014;**28**(11):3016-3045

[40] Leblanc M, Ouimet D, Pichette V. Dialysate leaks in peritoneal dialysis. Seminars in Dialysis. 2001;**14**(1):50-54

[41] Mital S, Fried LF, Piraino B. Bleeding complications associated with peritoneal dialysis catheter insertion. Peritoneal Dialysis International: Journal of the

International Society for Peritoneal Dialysis. 2004;**24**(5):478-480

[42] Chow KM, Wong KT, Szeto CC, Leung CB, Li PKT. Poor flow from Tenckhoff catheter. Hong Kong Journal of Nephrology. 2013;**15**(1):51-52

[43] Bakkaloglu SA, Borzych D, Soo Ha I, Serdaroglu E, Büscher R, Salas P, et al. Cardiac geometry in children receiving chronic peritoneal dialysis: Findings from the International Pediatric Peritoneal Dialysis Network (IPPN) registry. Clinical Journal of the American Society of Nephrology. 2011;**6**(8):1926-1933

[44] Honda M. The 1997 report of the Japanese National Registry data on pediatric peritoneal dialysis patients. Peritoneal Dialysis International: Journal of the International Society for Peritoneal Dialysis. 1999;**19**(Suppl. 2):S473-S478

[45] Shroff RC, Donald AE, Hiorns MP, Watson A, Feather S, Milford D, et al. Mineral metabolism and vascular damage in children on dialysis. Journal of the American Society of Nephrology : JASN. 2007;**18**(11):2996-3003

[46] Borzych-Duzalka D, Bilginer Y, Ha IS, Bak M, Rees L, Cano F, et al. Management of Anemia in children receiving chronic peritoneal dialysis. Journal of the American Society of Nephrology : JASN. 2013;**24**(4):665-676

[47] Pattaragarn A, Warady BA, Sabath RJ. Exercise capacity in pediatric patients with end-stage renal disease. Peritoneal Dialysis International: Journal of the International Society for Peritoneal Dialysis. 2004;**24**(3):274-280

[48] Di Zazzo G, Guzzo I, De Galasso L, Fortunato M, Leozappa G, Peruzzi L, et al. Anterior ischemic optical neuropathy in children on chronic peritoneal dialysis: Report of 7 cases. Peritoneal Dialysis International: Journal of the International Society for Peritoneal Dialysis. 2015;**35**(2):135-139

[49] Flynn JT, Kaelber DC, Baker-Smith CM, Blowey D, Carroll AE, Daniels SR, et al. Clinical practice guideline for screening and management of high blood pressure in children and adolescents. Pediatrics. 2017;**140**(3):e20171904

[50] KDIGO. Blood pressure management in children with CKD. Kidney International. 2012;**2**(Chapter 3):372-376

[51] Fischbach M, Warady BA. Peritoneal dialysis prescription in children: Bedside principles for optimal practice. Pediatric Nephrology. 2009;**24**(9):1633-1642

[52] Rousso S, Banh TM, Ackerman S, Piva E, Licht C, Harvey EA. Impact of fill volume on ultrafiltration with icodextrin in children on chronic peritoneal dialysis. Pediatric Nephrology. 2016;**31**(10):1673-1679

[53] Dart A, Feber J, Wong H, Filler G. Icodextrin re-absorption varies with age in children on automated peritoneal dialysis. Pediatric Nephrology. 2005;**20**(5):683-685

[54] Schaefer F, Borzych-Duzalka D, Warady B. Peritoneal dialysis prescription characteristics and outcomes in children: Analysis of the IPPN cohort. 2019. Available from: http://www.pedpd.org

[55] Fischbach M, Schmitt CP, Shroff R, Zaloszyc A, Warady BA. Increasing sodium removal on peritoneal dialysis: Applying dialysis mechanics to the peritoneal dialysis prescription. Kidney International. 2016;**89**(4):761-766

[56] Ha IS, Yap HK, Munarriz RL, Zambrano PH, Flynn JT, Bilge I, et al.

Risk factors for loss of residual renal function in children treated with chronic peritoneal dialysis. Kidney International. 2015;**88**(3):605-613

[57] Wuhl E, Trivelli A, Picca S, et al. Strict blood-pressure con trol and progression of renal failure in children. The New England Journal of Medicine. 2009;**361**(17):1639-1650

[58] Bakkaloglu SA, Wesseling-Perry K, Pereira RC, Gales B, Wang HJ, Elashoff RM, et al. Value of the new bone classification system in pediatric renal osteodystrophy. Clinical Journal of the American Society of Nephrology. 2010;**5**(10):1860-1866

[59] Schmitt CP, Borzych D, Nau B, Wühl E, Zurowska A, Schaefer F. Dialytic phosphate removal: A modifiable measure of dialysis efficacy in automated peritoneal dialysis. Peritoneal Dialysis International : Journal of the International Society for Peritoneal Dialysis. 2009;**29**(4):465-471

[60] Daugirdas JT, Hanna MG, Becker-Cohen R, Langman CB. Dose of dialysis based on body surface area is markedly less in younger children than in older adolescents. Clinical Journal of the American Society of Nephrology. 2010;**5**(5):821-827

[61] Hanson CS, Gutman T, Craig JC, Bernays S, Raman G, Zhang Y, et al. Identifying important outcomes for young people with CKD and their caregivers: A nominal group technique study. American Journal of Kidney Diseases. 2019;**74**(1):82-94

[62] On behalf of the Song-Kids Investigators, Tong A, Samuel S, Zappitelli M, Dart A, Furth S, et al. Standardised outcomes in nephrology—Children and adolescents (SONG-kids): A protocol for establishing a core outcome set for children with chronic kidney disease. Trials. 2016;**17**(1):401

[63] Bernardini J, Price V, Figueiredo A. International Society for Peritoneal Dialysis (ISPD) nursing liaison Committee. Peritoneal dialysis patient training, 2006. Peritoneal Dialysis International: Journal of the International Society for Peritoneal Dialysis. 2006;**26**(6):625-632

[64] Bernardini J, Price V, Figueiredo A, Riemann A, Leung D. International survey of peritoneal dialysis training programs. Peritoneal Dialysis International: Journal of the International Society for Peritoneal Dialysis. 2006;**26**(6):658-663

[65] Coles G, Uttley L. Recommendations of the International Society for Peritoneal Dialysis for training requirements of nephrology trainees and nurses. Peritoneal Dialysis International. 1994;**14**(2):117-120

[66] Bender FH, Bernardini J, Piraino B. Prevention of infectious complications in peritoneal dialysis: Best demonstrated practices. Kidney International. 2006;**70**:S44-S54

[67] Miller TE, Findon G. Touch contamination of connection devices in peritoneal dialysis–A quantitative microbiologic analysis. Peritoneal Dialysis International: Journal of the International Society for Peritoneal Dialysis. 1997;**17**(6):560-567

[68] Watson AR, Gartland C. European paediatric peritoneal dialysis working group. Guidelines by an ad hoc European Committee for Elective Chronic Peritoneal Dialysis in Pediatric patients. Peritoneal Dialysis International: Journal of the International Society for Peritoneal Dialysis. 2001;**21**(3):240-244

[69] Sethna CB, Bryant K, Munshi R, Warady BA, Richardson T, Lawlor J, et al. Risk factors for and outcomes of catheter-associated peritonitis in children: The SCOPE collaborative. Clinical Journal of the American Society of Nephrology. 2016;**11**(9):1590-1596

[70] Redpath Mahon A, Neu AM. A contemporary approach to the prevention of peritoneal dialysis-related peritonitis in children: The role of improvement science. Pediatric Nephrology. 2017;**32**(8):1331-1341

[71] KDIGO. Clinical practice guideline for lipid Management in Chronic Kidney Disease. Kidney International. 2013;(Supplement 3):259-305

[72] Shroff R, Wan M, Nagler EV, Bakkaloğlu S, Cozzolino M, Bacchetta J, et al. Clinical practice recommendations for treatment with active vitamin D analogues in children with chronic kidney disease stages 2-5 and on dialysis. Nephrology, Dialysis, Transplantation. 2017;**32**(7):1114-1127

[73] Shroff R, Wan M, Nagler EV, Bakkaloğlu S, Fischer DC, Bishop N, et al. Clinical practice recommendations for native vitamin D therapy in children with chronic kidney disease stages 2-5 and on dialysis. Nephrology, Dialysis, Transplantation. 2017;**32**(7):1098-1113

[74] Sutherland SM, Byrnes JJ, Kothari M, Longhurst CA, Dutta S, Garcia P, et al. AKI in hospitalized children: Comparing the pRIFLE, AKIN, and KDIGO definitions. Clinical Journal of the American Society of Nephrology. 2015;**10**(4):554-561

[75] Jetton JG, Boohaker LJ, Sethi SK, Wazir S, Rohatgi S, Soranno DE, et al. Incidence and outcomes of neonatal acute kidney injury (AWAKEN): A multicentre, multinational, observational cohort study. The Lancet. Child & Adolescent Health. 2017;**1**(3):184-194

[76] Kaddourah A, Basu RK, Bagshaw SM, Goldstein SL. Epidemiology of acute kidney injury in critically ill children and young adults. The New England Journal of Medicine. 2017;**376**(1):11-20

[77] McGregor TL, Jones DP, Wang L, Danciu I, Bridges BC, Fleming GM, et al. Acute kidney injury incidence in noncritically ill hospitalized children, adolescents, and young adults: A retrospective observational study. American Journal of Kidney Diseases. 2016;**67**(3):384-390

[78] Olowu WA, Niang A, Osafo C, Ashuntantang G, Arogundade FA, Porter J, et al. Outcomes of acute kidney injury in children and adults in sub-Saharan Africa: A systematic review. The Lancet Global Health. 2016;**4**(4):e242-e250

[79] Raina R, Chauvin AM, Bunchman T, Askenazi D, Deep A, Ensley MJ, et al. Treatment of AKI in developing and developed countries: An international survey of pediatric dialysis modalities. PLoS One. 2017;**12**(5):e0178233

[80] For the ESCAPE Network, Guzzo I, De Galasso L, Mir S, Bulut IK, Jankauskiene A, et al. Acute dialysis in children: Results of a European survey. Journal of Nephrology. 2019;**32**(3):445-451

[81] Ao X, Zhong Y, Xhe Y, Marshall MR, Feng T, Ping NJ, et al. Acute peritoneal dialysis system for neonates with acute kidney injury requiring renal replacement therapy: A case series. Peritoneal Dialysis International: Journal of the International Society for Peritoneal Dialysis. 2018;**38**(2_Suppl.):45-52

[82] Burgmaier K, Hackl A, Ehren R, Kribs A, Burgmaier M, Weber LT, et al. Peritoneal dialysis in extremely and very low-birth-weight infants. Peritoneal Dialysis International: Journal of the International Society for Peritoneal Dialysis. 2020;**40**(2):233-236

[83] Stojanović VD, Bukarica SS, Antić JB, Doronjski AD. Peritoneal dialysis in very low birth weight neonates. Peritoneal Dialysis International: Journal of the International Society for Peritoneal Dialysis. 2017;**37**(4):389-396

[84] Barhight MF, Soranno D, Faubel S, Gist KM. Fluid management with peritoneal dialysis after pediatric cardiac surgery. World Journal for Pediatric & Congenital Heart Surgery. 2018;**9**(6):696-704

[85] Vasudevan A, Phadke K, Yap HK. Peritoneal dialysis for the management of pediatric patients with acute kidney injury. Pediatric Nephrology. 2017;**32**:1145-1156

[86] Nourse P, Cullis B, Finkelstein F, Numanoglu A, Warady B, Antwi S, et al. ISPD guidelines for peritoneal dialysis in acute kidney injury: 2020 update (paediatrics). Peritoneal Dialysis International: Journal of the International Society for Peritoneal Dialysis. 2021;**41**(2):139-157

[87] Grading quality of evidence and strength of recommendations. BMJ. 2004;**328**(7454):1490

[88] Reznik VM, Randolph G, Collins CM, Peterson BM, Lemire JM, Mendoza SA. Cost analysis of dialysis modalities for pediatric acute renal failure. Peritoneal Dialysis International: Journal of the International Society for Peritoneal Dialysis. 1993;**13**(4):311-313

[89] Flynn JT. Choice of dialysis modality for management of pediatric acute renal failure. Pediatric Nephrology. 2002;**17**(1):61-69

[90] George J, Varma S, Kumar S, Thomas J, Gopi S, Pisharody R. Comparing continuous venovenous hemodiafiltration and peritoneal dialysis in critically ill patients with acute kidney injury: A pilot study. Peritoneal Dialysis International: Journal of the International Society for Peritoneal Dialysis. 2011;**31**(4):422-429

[91] Golej J, Kitzmueller E, Hermon M, Boigner H, Burda G, Trittenwein G. Low-volume peritoneal dialysis in 116 neonatal and paediatric critical care patients. European Journal of Pediatrics. 2002;**161**(7):385-389

[92] Flynn JT, Kershaw DB, Smoyer WE, Brophy PD, McBryde KD, Bunchman TE. Peritoneal dialysis for management of pediatric acute renal failure. Peritoneal Dialysis International: Journal of the International Society for Peritoneal Dialysis. 2001;**21**(4):390-394

[93] Fleming F, Bohn D, Edwards H, Cox P, Geary D, McCrindle BW, et al. Renal replacement therapy after repair of congenital heart disease in children. The Journal of Thoracic and Cardiovascular Surgery. 1995;**109**(2):322-331

[94] Basu B, Mahapatra TKS, Roy B, Schaefer F. Efficacy and outcomes of continuous peritoneal dialysis versus daily intermittent hemodialysis in pediatric acute kidney injury. Pediatric Nephrology. 2016;**31**(10):1681-1689

[95] Krause I, Herman N, Cleper R, Fraser A, Davidovits M. Impact of dialysis type on outcome of acute renal failure in children: A single-center experience. The Israel

Medical Association Journal: IMAJ. 2011;**13**(3):153-156

[96] Kwiatkowski DM, Goldstein SL, Cooper DS, Nelson DP, Morales DLS, Krawczeski CD. Peritoneal dialysis vs furosemide for prevention of fluid overload in infants after cardiac surgery: A randomized clinical trial. JAMA Pediatrics. 2017;**171**(4):357

[97] Pedersen KR, Hjortdal VE, Christensen S, Pedersen J, Hjortholm K, Larsen SH, et al. Clinical outcome in children with acute renal failure treated with peritoneal dialysis after surgery for congenital heart disease. Kidney International. 2008;**73**:S81-S86

[98] Chadha V, Warady BA, Blowey DL, Simckes AM, Alon US. Tenckhoff catheters prove superior to cook catheters in pediatric acute peritoneal dialysis. American Journal of Kidney Diseases. 2000;**35**(6):1111-1116

[99] Wong SN, Geary DF. Comparison of temporary and permanent catheters for acute peritoneal dialysis. Archives of Disease in Childhood. 1988;**63**(7):827-831

[100] Stack M, Price N, Ronaldson J, Prestidge C, Wong W, Kara T. Laparoscopic versus open peritoneal dialysis catheter insertion for the management of pediatric acute kidney injury. Pediatric Nephrology. 2016;**31**(2):297-303

[101] LaPlant MB, Saltzman DA, Segura BJ, Acton RD, Feltis BA, Hess DJ. Peritoneal dialysis catheter placement, outcomes and complications. Pediatric Surgery International. 2018;**34**(11):1239-1244

[102] Murala JSK, Singappuli K, Provenzano SC, Nunn G. Techniques of inserting peritoneal dialysis catheters in neonates and infants undergoing open heart surgery. The Journal of Thoracic and Cardiovascular Surgery. 2010;**139**(2):503-505

[103] Swan P, Darwish A, Elbarbary M, Halees ZA. The safety of peritoneal drainage and dialysis after cardiopulmonary bypass in children. The Journal of Thoracic and Cardiovascular Surgery. 1997;**114**(4):688-689

[104] Sorof JM, Stromberg D, Brewer ED, Feltes TF, Fraser CD Jr. Early initiation of peritoneal dialysis after surgical repair of congenital heart disease. Pediatric Nephrology. 1999;**13**(8):641-645

[105] Gong WK, Tan TH, Foong PP, Murugasu B, Yap HK. Eighteen years experience in pediatric acute dialysis: Analysis of predictors of outcome. Pediatric Nephrology. 2001;**16**(3):212-215

[106] Bunchman TE. Acute peritoneal dialysis access in infant renal failure. Peritoneal Dialysis International: Journal of the International Society for Peritoneal Dialysis. 1996;**16**(Suppl. 1):S509-S511

[107] Kohli HS, Barkataky A, Kumar RSV, Sud K, Jha V, Gupta KL, et al. Peritoneal dialysis for acute renal failure in infants: A comparison of three types of peritoneal access. Renal Failure. 1997;**19**(1):165-170

[108] Abdelraheem M, Ali ET, Osman R, Ellidir R, Bushara A, Hussein R, et al. Outcome of acute kidney injury in Sudanese children — An experience from a sub-Saharan African unit. Peritoneal Dialysis International: Journal of the International Society for Peritoneal Dialysis. 2014;**34**(5):526-533

[109] Kiernan L, Kliger A, Gorban-Brennan N, Juergensen P, Tesin D, Vonesh E, et al. Comparison of continuous ambulatory peritoneal

dialysis-related infections with different « Y-tubing » exchange systems. Journal of the American Society of Nephrology : JASN. 1995;**5**(10):1835-1838

[110] Valeri A, Radhakrishnan J, Vernocchi L, Carmichael LD, Stern L. The epidemiology of peritonitis in acute peritoneal dialysis: A comparison between open- and closed-drainage systems. American Journal of Kidney Diseases. 1993;**21**(3):300-309

[111] Ansari N. Peritoneal dialysis in renal replacement therapy for patients with acute kidney injury. International Journal of Nephrology. 2011;**2011**:1-10

[112] Ponce D, Berbel MN, Regina De Goes C, Almeida CTP, Balbi AL. High-volume peritoneal dialysis in acute kidney injury: Indications and limitations. Clinical Journal of the American Society of Nephrology. 2012;**7**(6):887-894

[113] Ponce D, Balbi AL, Amerling R. Advances in peritoneal dialysis in acute kidney injury. Blood Purification. 2012;**34**(2):107-116

[114] Krediet RT. The physiology of peritoneal solute, water, and lymphatic transport. In: Khanna R, Krediet RT, editors. Nolph and Gokal's textbook of peritoneal dialysis. 3rd edn. New York, NY: Springer; 2009. pp. 137-172

[115] Brophy PD, Yap HK, Alexander SR. Acute kidney injury: Diagnosis and treatment with peritoneal dialysis, hemodialysis, and CRRT. Pediatric Dialysis. 2012;**2**:697-736

[116] Bai ZG, Yang K, Tian JH, et al. Bicarbonate versus lactate solutions for acute peritoneal dialysis. Cochrane Database of Systematic Reviews. 2014;**2014**(7):1-14, CD007034

[117] Morgenstern BZ. Equilibration testing: Close, but not quite right. Pediatric Nephrology (Berlin, Germany). 1993;**7**(3):290-291

[118] Bunchman TE, Meldrum MK, Meliones JE, Sedman AB, Walters MB, Kershaw DB. Pulmonary function variation in ventilator dependent critically ill infants on peritoneal dialysis. Advances in Peritoneal Dialysis. Conference on Peritoneal Dialysis. 1992;**8**:75-78

[119] Fischbach M. Peritoneal dialysis prescription for neonates. Peritoneal Dialysis International: Journal of the International Society for Peritoneal Dialysis. 1996;**16**(Suppl. 1):S512-S514

[120] Selewski DT, Goldstein SL. The role of fluid overload in the prediction of outcome in acute kidney injury. Pediatric Nephrology. 2018;**33**(1):13-24

[121] Raaijmakers R, Schröder CH, Gajjar P, Argent A, Nourse P. Continuous flow peritoneal dialysis: First experience in children with acute renal failure. Clinical Journal of the American Society of Nephrology. 2011;**6**(2):311-318

[122] Nourse P, Sinclair G, Gajjar P, Du Plessis M, Argent AC. Continuous flow peritoneal dialysis (CFPD) improves ultrafiltration in children with acute kidney injury on conventional PD using a 4.25% dextrose solution. Pediatric Nephrology. 2016;**31**(7):1137-1143

[123] Yu JE, Park MS, Pai KS. Acute peritoneal dialysis in very low birth weight neonates using a vascular catheter. Pediatric Nephrology. 2010;**25**(2):367-371

[124] Nepfumbada M, Naicker E, Bhimma R. Peritoneal infections in children undergoing acute peritoneal dialysis at a tertiary/quaternary central

Hospital in Kwazulu-Natal, South Africa. Peritoneal Dialysis International: Journal of the International Society for Peritoneal Dialysis. 2018;**38**(6):413-418

[125] Mishra OP, Gupta AK, Pooniya V, Prasad R, Tiwary NK, Schaefer F. Peritoneal dialysis in children with acute kidney injury: A developing country experience. Peritoneal Dialysis International: Journal of the International Society for Peritoneal Dialysis. 2012;**32**(4):431-436

[126] McCulloch MI, Nourse P, Argent AC. Use of locally prepared peritoneal dialysis (PD) fluid for acute PD in children and infants in Africa. Peritoneal Dialysis International: Journal of the International Society for Peritoneal Dialysis. 2020;**40**(5):441-445

[127] Vande Walle J, Raes A, Castillo D, Lutz-Dettinger N, Dejaegher A. New perspectives for PD in acute renal failure related to new catheter techniques and introduction of APD. Advances in Peritoneal Dialysis. Conference on Peritoneal Dialysis. 1997;**13**:190-194

[128] Auron A, Warady BA, Simon S, Blowey DL, Srivastava T, Musharaf G, et al. Use of the multipurpose drainage catheter for the provision of acute peritoneal dialysis in infants and children. American Journal of Kidney Diseases. 2007;**49**(5):650-655

[129] Santos CR, Branco PQ, Gaspar A, Bruges M, Anjos R, Gonçalves MS, et al. Use of peritoneal dialysis after surgery for congenital heart disease in children. Peritoneal Dialysis International: Journal of the International Society for Peritoneal Dialysis. 2012;**32**(3):273-279

[130] Borzych-Duzalka D, Aki TF, Azocar M, White C, Harvey E, Mir S, et al. Peritoneal dialysis access revision in children: Causes, interventions, and outcomes. Clinical Journal of the American Society of Nephrology. 2017;**12**(1):105-112

[131] Crabtree JH, Shrestha BM, Chow KM, Figueiredo AE, Povlsen JV, Wilkie M, et al. Creating and maintaining optimal peritoneal dialysis access in the adult patient: 2019 update. Peritoneal Dialysis International: Journal of the International Society for Peritoneal Dialysis. 2019;**39**(5):414-436

[132] Gabriel DP, Caramori JT, Martim LC, Barretti P, Balbi AL. High volume peritoneal dialysis vs daily hemodialysis: A randomized, controlled trial in patients with acute kidney injury. Kidney International. 2008;**73**:S87-S93

[133] Góes CR, Berbel MN, Balbi AL, Ponce D. Metabolic implications of peritoneal dialysis in patients with acute kidney injury. Peritoneal Dialysis International: Journal of the International Society for Peritoneal Dialysis. 2013;**33**(6):635-645

Chapter 6

Peritoneal Dialysis in Paediatric Acute Kidney Injury in Intensive Care Units: Prescription and Management

Djamila Djahida Batouche, Djilali Batouche, Zakaria-Zoheir Addou, Dalila Boumendil and Fatima Souhila Bouchama

Abstract

Acute kidney injury (AKI) is defined by a rapid decrease in glomerular filtration rate, leading to disruption of physiological functions, including impaired excretion of nitrogenous waste products, hydroelectrolytic disorders, and disturbance of acid-base balance. AKI is a major contributor to morbidity and mortality in severely affected infants and children, and its treatment, apart from symptomatic, etiological treatment, involves renal replacement therapy (intermittent haemodialysis, haemodialfiltration, haemofiltration, and peritoneal dialysis). In paediatric intensive care unit, emergency peritoneal dialysis (PD) is often the only possible technique for renal replacement therapy. It is easy to set up by the intensive care anaesthetist, or paediatric surgeon and uses the mechanisms of diffusion and osmosis (ultrafiltration). The anatomical properties of the peritoneum enable water and solute exchange. Solutions in bag form are available in isotonic or hypertonic concentrations, and their use depends on the clinical indications. PD has many advantages over other dialysis techniques, but there are some complications inherent in PD that need to be addressed by therapeutic protocols.

Keywords: continuous peritoneal dialysis, paediatric emergency, flexible catheter, solutions, intraperitoneal exchanges

1. Introduction

1.1 Acute kidney injury

In 2004, the term acute renal failure (ARF) was replaced by acute kidney injury (AKI), which better expresses the fact that it is a set of symptoms associated with sudden renal failure. The syndrome is characterised by a reduction in glomerular filtration rate (GFR), retention of urea and other metabolic products such as uric acid and ammonia, and dysregulation of extracellular volume and electrolytes [1–3]. AKI is therefore a syndrome with varied manifestations and not a disease in the strict sense.

AKI is an important factor contributing to morbidity and mortality in severely affected infants and children [4, 5].

Since 2007, four essential definitions for AKI in children have been published: [6–9] see (**Table 1**).

The Paediatric Risk Injury Failure Loss ESRD (pRIFLE) criteria. In parallel with the pRIFLE work, the Acute Kidney Injury Network (AKIN) published a consensus statement on acute kidney injury (AKI).

In 2012, the Kidney Disease Improving Global Outcome (KDIGO) definition was published. The Paediatric Reference change value Optimised for AKI (pROCK) definition was adopted in paediatrics in 2018 from a multicentre study in hospitalised children in multicentre China as creatinine increase beyond RCV of creatinine, which was estimated as the greater of 20 μmol/L or 30% of the initial creatinine level. pROCK It is less sensitive for the detection of AKI but more specific outperformed KDIGO and pRIFLE in predicting the mortality risk especially in children requiring intensive care.

Definitions and comparisons have been difficult between studies in the literature, resulting in a wide range of citations, epidemiologies, morbidities, and mortality rates [10].

Classification	Staging creatinine	Creatinine criteria	Urine output criteria
pRIFLE	Risk eGFR	decreased by ≥25%	0.5 mL/kg/hr. for 8 hr
	Injury	eGFR decreased by ≥50%	0.5 mL/kg/hr. for 16 h
	Failure	eGFR decreased by ≥75% (or < 35 mL/min/1.73 m^2)	0.3 mL/kg/hr. for 24 hr. or anuria for 12
	Loss	Persistent failure >4 wk	
	ESRD	ESRD persistent failure >3 mo	
AKIN	1	Increase in creatinine of ≥50% or an absolute increase in creatinine of 0.3 mg/dL over 48-hr period	
	2	Increase in creatinine of ≥100%	
	3	Increase in creatinine of ≥200%	
KDIGO	1	SCr rise ≥0.3 mg/dL within 48 hr. or an increase in creatinine of≥50% within 7 day	>0.5 and ≤ 1 mL/kg/hr
	2	Increase in creatinine of ≥100%	>0.3 and ≤ 0.5 mL/kg/h
	3	Increase in creatinine of ≥200% or SCr ≥4 mg/dL or receipt of dialysis or eGFR<35 mL/min/1.73 m^2	≤ 0.3 mL/kg/hr

AKIN, Acute Kidney Injury Network; eGFR, estimated glomerular filtration rate; ESRD, end-stage renal disease; KDIGO, Kidney Disease: Improving Global Outcomes; pRIFLE, paediatric risk, injury, failure, loss of kidney function, and end-stage kidney disease; SCr, serum creatinine.

Table 1.
Paediatric acute kidney injury definitions.

In the newborn, there is no consensus definition for AKI. It was suggested that a classification AKI KDIGO for neonates and infants <120 days old [11]:

serum creatinine increase ≥0.3 mg/dL (26.5 mcmol/L) within 48 hours OR

- Stage 1 serum creatinine increase ≥1.5–1.9 times reference serum creatinine within 7 days, defined as the lowest previous serum creatinine value urine output <0.5 mL/kg/hour for 6–12 hours

- Stage 2, either of serum creatinine increase ≥2–2.9 times reference serum creatinine (defined as the lowest previous serum creatinine value) urine output <0.5 mL/kg/hour for ≥12 hours

- Stage 3, any of serum creatinine increase ≥3 times reference serum creatinine (defined as the lowest previous serum creatinine value) serum creatinine ≥2.5 mg/dL, which represents glomerular filtration rate < 10 mL/minute/1.73 m^2 initiation of renal replacement therapy

  urine output <0.3 mL/kg/hour for ≥24 hours

  anuria for ≥12 hours

In the most severe cases, renal replacement therapy (RRT) is initiated to supplement renal function.

Several paediatric publications use peritoneal dialysis as one of the other RRT [12–14].

PD in emergency setting of the paediatric intensive care unit remains the only possible technique for RRT in infants, based on the experience of nursing staff and the unavailability of RRT equipment adapted to the child's weight because of the difficulties of vascular access, the risk of bleeding, and hypotension in an extracorporeal circulation [15–18].

We will focus solely on PD in children with AKI while discussing prescription methods, the complications of PD, and how to manage them.

1.2 Anatomy and physiology of peritoneal membrane

The peritoneum is composed of two adjacent layers: the parietal peritoneum which adheres to the anterior abdominal wall and which covers behind the retro peritoneum and the peritoneum visceral which totally or partially covers the abdominal organs.

It presents folds:

- Ligaments, means of fixing organs, without a main vascular pedicle within them;

- Theomentums that have a free edge;

- Themesos that contain the main vascular pedicle of the organ.

Between the two layers of the parietal and visceral peritoneum, we find the peritoneal cavity, which contains a thin layer of lubricating fluid, thus preventing friction during the movements of the abdominal organs. This liquid less than 100 ml is produced by the peritoneal layers and is resorbed by lymphatic plexuses that are particularly numerous at the level of the lower surface of the right diaphragm. About 100 mL of a liquid formed from an ultrafiltrate of the peritoneum.

The peritoneal membrane successively comprises, from the blood to the peritoneal dialysate, the basement membrane of the peritoneal capillaries, the supporting connective tissue, the submesothelial basement membrane, and the monolayer of mesothelial cells.

The peritoneal membrane surface area is roughly equal to the body surface area.

PD does not require an extracorporeal blood circuit, and the exchanges between the blood and the dialysis solution (infused into the peritoneal cavity by a catheter) take place through the walls of the rich vascular network of the peritoneal membrane, according to the concentration gradients.

Peritoneal exchanges are based on two fundamental principles: diffusion (dialysis) and convection (ultrafiltration), as well as the three-pore model [19].

Transfer by diffusion occurs under the influence of a concentration gradient: urea, creatinine, calcium, phosphorus, and other plasma waste substances are gradually transferred into the dialysis fluid which is devoid of them, while the transfer is from the dialysis fluid to the blood for glucose, the buffer anion (lactate or bicarbonate), and calcium.

Ultrafiltration: Net ultrafiltration is achieved clinically by creating an osmotic pressure gradient such as glycerol, amino acids, glucose polymers, or icodextrin. Solutes present in body fluids can be carried away by the bulk solvent flow, even in the absence of a concentration difference for net diffusion, which contributes to the overall clearance of solutes. This contribution to net solute clearance has been termed 'convection'.

Three-pore model: [19].

There are three types of pore of different sizes in the endothelium of peritoneal capillaries.

The small, intercellular pores are where water and low-molecular-weight molecules such as electrolytes, urea, creatinine, and glucose pass through.

The ultra-small pores, which are the most numerous, are characterised by transcellular channels or aquaporins. They transport only free water, thus diluting the dialysate with a reduction in the initial sodium concentration and transfer from the plasma by concentration gradient or sodium sieving.

The large pores, which are few in number, allow large substances such as proteins and glucose polymers (icodextrin) to pass through the intercellular spaces.

This three-pore model makes it possible to explain peritoneal transfer by convection according to osmotic pressure of crystalloid or colloid origin and according to intraperitoneal hydrostatic pressure.

1.3 Peritoneal dialysis as a treatment for acute kidney injury

Despite the increasing importance of continuous haemofiltration techniques, PD is the most common and simplest method of ensuring the elimination of solutes and water in severe AKI, and has a major role to play in the management of AKI, especially in paediatric units where access to other extra-renal purification techniques is difficult or even impossible. It is very easy to perform in the patient's bed or in the operating theatre and does not require vascular access.

Acute PD is currently the best treatment modality for primary or complicated kidney disease-causing AKI.: The commonest cause was hypoperfusion, haemolytic-uremic syndrome (HUS), [20], hypernatremic dehydration [21, 22], sepsis infection [23, 24], volume depletion, hypoxia ischemia, intrinsic renal disease, cardiogenic shock, post-surgical [25], and malaria in Africa [26]; peritoneal dialysis was the early treatment for children after cardiac surgery [27]. All AKI secondary to nephrotoxicity and poisoning were treated by PD in children in intensive care [23, 28].

During the COVID-19 pandemic, telemedicine was used to guide patients treated with chronic peritoneal dialysis in adults and has potential to improve patient care quality.

It is safety measures on how to protect PD patients and médical staffs.

The pandemic affected very few children during the first decade; however, some children developed acute kidney injury (AKI) with paediatric multisystem inflammatory syndrome (pMIS), and PD has attracted renewed interest in resource-limited countries, with the advantages of cost-effectiveness, ease of training, and reduced electricity and water requirements making PD the optimal form of therapy.

In both the adult and paediatric populations, there is sufficient evidence to demonstrate that peritoneal dialysis is as effective as other forms of RRT [29–32].

2. Advantages of acute peritoneal dialysis

PD is not associated with dialysis imbalance syndrome and may be more appropriate for patients with elevated intracranial pressure. Vascular access is not required for PD and has a significant advantage in small children where insertion of a peritoneal catheter is often easier than insertion of a dialysis catheter, especially in neonates [33].

PD makes it possible to preserve residual diuresis, and intraperitoneal exchanges ensure good haemodynamic tolerance [33].

In a prospective study, at Week 4 of admission or discharge, early initiation of PD in patients with SA-AKI was associated with early renal recovery and higher eGFR [24].

PD offers other advantages such as: the absence of extracorporeal circulation with its inherent risks (gas embolism, central catheter infection, and hypovolaemia) and the possibility of following a freer diet (especially in the catabolic phase), and it avoids anticoagulation and is inexpensive [3]. In infants, protection of the venous outlets is a crucial factor, especially if there is a high risk of progression to chronic kidney failure.

3. Limitations associated with acute peritoneal dialysis

PD uses the peritoneum as

1. Means of convection and ultrafiltration, so this peritoneum must be intact and free of contraindications to the placement of the peritoneal dialysis catheter, such as

   Recent surgery, peritoneal drains in place, omphalocele, laparoschisis or diaphragmatic hernia in children, fungal peritonitis peritonitis, and abdominal compartment syndrome;

   Even if PD remains effective, it is not without mechanical, infectious, and metabolic complications, which will be detailed in the chapter on complications of peritoneal dialysis.

2. It is more delicate in the event of respiratory distress and makes intubation and support by assisted ventilation necessary, especially in infants and newborns, due to an increase in abdominal volume during the dialysate infusion phase, thus resulting in insufficient ultrafiltration [34].

3. The time required to achieve satisfactory metabolic control and adequate volume control using PD makes this technique unsuitable for life-threatening emergencies—It is not the best modality for RRT in patients with threatening hyperkalaemia and those with hypercatabolism with a high azotemia load as this can only be achieved after 24 hours of dialysis [35]

4. In PD, clearance is limited by the flow rate of the dialysate, the permeability of the membrane, and the surface area coefficient (KoA). In PD, clearance is limited by dialysate flow membrane [36]

PD is less effective than haemodialysis or CRRT in children with inborn errors of metabolism (IEM), such as hyperammoniaemia, where neurological outcome is correlated with the speed and normalisation of blood urea treatment [37].

3.1 Peritoneal dialysis compared with other renal replacement therapy techniques

Observational studies comparing the modalities showed no difference in mortality between children treated with PD and those receiving CRRT to treat AKI.

A retrospective study by Fleming et al. [38] of 34 children who had undergone cardiac surgery showed that CRRT was associated with better fluid control and nutritional support than PD, but there was no significant difference in mortality rates, similarly in Flynn's series [3].

Comparing the safety of PD versus intermittent haemodialysis, a retrospective study by Basu et al. [25] found that the risk of death in patients treated with HD was 75% higher than in patients treated with PD. The children treated with HD in this study experienced frequent episodes of hypotension during treatment, and a risk analysis of the causes of death suggested that fluid and electrolyte changes were possible causes.

Krause et al. [39] found that intermittent HD was associated with a significantly better outcome than PD or haemodiafiltration (HDF) in another retrospective study of 115 children requiring dialysis for AKI. In this study, patients treated with IHD and PD were critical and placed on haemodynamic support, and the number of children treated with PD was significantly greater than in the other renal replacement therapies.

Gabriel et al. [40] then randomised 60 patients between acute high-volume PD and daily haemodialysis. There was no significant difference in terms of mortality.

However, recovery of renal function was observed 3 days earlier in the PD group.

In both the adult and paediatric populations, there is sufficient evidence to demonstrate that peritoneal dialysis is as effective as other forms of renal replacement. Recommendation 1B in adults and 1C in paediatrics, according to which PD is suitable for the treatment of AKI in all settings [41, 42].

4. Indications for acute peritoneal dialysis in children

PD can be carried out as an emergency treatment for AKI with no other organ failure.

- Hyperkalaemia, severe metabolic acidosis, and fluid overload, after failure of medical treatment.
- Risk of progression to kidney failure [43, 44]
- Renal indications and no renal indications of peritoneal dialysis in AKI are summarised in (**Table 2**) adapted by Ansari [45].

5. Efficiency of acute peritoneal dialysis

Numerous case series and randomised trials of PD in AKI demonstrate rapid correction of hyperkalaemia, acidosis, and fluid overload, usually returning to normal levels within 24–48 hours [46, 47].

Cullis et al. [48] recommend that in patients with AKI, a weekly Kt/V of 2.1 may be acceptable.

At present, there are no data correlating clearance and outcome in children undergoing acute PD, so no target dialysis dose can be set. In two paediatric studies of ARF of various aetiologies, the use of a filling volume of 20 ml/kg and a contact time of 60 minutes resulted in a mean weekly creatinine clearance of 75 l/week/1.73m^2.

McNiece et al. [49] measured clearance in five neonates undergoing cardiac surgery using a filling volume of 10 ml/kg and a contact time of 20 minutes. The median weekly creatinine clearance was 74 l/week/1.73 m^2, and the median Kt/V was 4.84.

Finally, Ricci et al. [50] determined that the creatinine clearance of 20 neonates post-cardiac surgery was 34 l/week/1.73 m^2 using a PD filling volume of 10 ml/kg and variable contact times, irrespective of haemodynamic status or drug vasopressor support.

These studies show that despite the low filling volumes and frequent cycles used in paediatrics, the clearances obtained are higher than those recommended in the adult literature [41].

Acute PD is an effective and reliable alternative to renal replacement therapy, particularly for reducing BUN and K+ levels in preterm neonates with AKI, in a retrospective study conducted by Xing et al. [51] including 21 preterm neonates who

Renal indications of peritoneal dialysis in AKI	Nonrenal indications
1. RRT in the treatment of AKI in children	1. Acute pancreatitis
2. Hemodynamically unstable patients	2. Clinically significant hypothermia or hyperthermia
3. The presence of bleeding diathesis or haemorragic conditions contraindicating placement of vascular access for haemodialysis or anticoagulation	3. Refractory heart failure
4. Patients with difficult vascular access placement	4. Liver failure
5. Removal of high molecular weight toxins (10 kD)	5. Infusion of drugs and nutrients as a supportive therapy in critically ill patients

Table 2.
Indications of peritoneal dialysis.

underwent APD in a neonatal intensive care unit (NICU) in Peking University Third Hospital. The median duration of PD was 3 days (range, 1 hour-20 days). Compared with the period before PD, blood urea nitrogen (BUN) and serum K+ levels decreased significantly after PD ($P < 0.05$). Oedema disappeared in 77.8% (n = 14/18) of patients, and 42.9% (n = 9/21) of patients regained normal urine output.

6. Strategies to improve dialysis efficiency in acute peritoneal dialysis

The strategy for improving the effectiveness of peritoneal dialysis will depend on several factors:

6.1 Choice of catheter

The common types of catheters used in acute PD are the rigid stylet catheter, Tenckhoff catheter, and Cook (Cook Medical Inc., Bloomington, IN) Teflon rigid catheter. The semi-rigid catheter can be inserted at the patient's bedside by a resuscitator under local anaesthetic, avoiding the need for a general anaesthetic.

The literature shows the effectiveness of the Tenckhoff catheter compared with other catheters [52].

6.2 Access to the peritoneal cavity

In emergency conditions, the catheter can be placed using a trocar and under peritoneoscopic control, although this technique requires general anaesthesia.

Laparoscopic catheter placement is successfully employed in children in many centres [53–55]. However, catheter placement for long-term peritoneal dialysis treatment is best performed surgically, under rigorous aseptic conditions, by a trained and motivated operator.

The most commonly used catheter entry route is paramedian, slightly below the level of the umbilicus, most often on the right side, the choice being guided by the patient's build.

Before the catheter is inserted, it is essential to reassure the child's parents and get them to sign an informed consent form, explaining the principle of the procedure and how it will be carried out. The catheter is usually inserted under general anaesthetic.

After carefully disinfecting the skin of the abdomen, an incision a few centimetres long is made through the fibres of the rectus abdominis, which are gently pulled apart to just the right length.

The catheter is inserted under visual control using a metal guide, the tip of the catheter being pushed into the lower part of the pelvic cavity, at the level of the cul de sac of Douglas. The tip of the catheter is then in contact with the lateral surface of the rectum. Once the catheter is firmly in place, the first Dacron® flange is fixed at a 45° angle in the peritoneal suture, which is then carefully closed around the catheter and its flange.

A tunnel is then created under the skin, allowing the catheter to pass subcutaneously. The second Dacron® flange is carefully fixed a few centimetres before the exit port, to prevent extrusion.

Check that the catheter is working properly immediately after insertion: after instilling approximately 1 litre of sterile isotonic solution, the liquid should return easily and be perfectly clear.

However, catheter malfunction, that is difficulty in draining the solution introduced into the peritoneal cavity, is not uncommon at the time of insertion. In this case, the position of the catheter should be checked by X-ray of the abdomen: when the peritoneal segment of the catheter has moved and is no longer resting in the cul de sac of Douglas, it may be necessary to intervene surgically to put it back in the correct position.

6.3 Peritoneal dialysis fluid and method of fluid delivery

Although the peritoneal membrane is biocompatible and natural, conventional dialysate fluids containing dextrose can alter the functionality of the peritoneal membrane due to glucose degradation products and the use of lactate as a buffer.

Fischbach et al. [56] demonstrated in children undergoing chronic dialysis that the use of a bicarbonate-lactate buffer gave good results in terms of a reduction in abdominal pressure during filling, alleviation of abdominal pain, and therefore good integrity of peritoneal function.

The composition of the dialysate fluid is summarised (**Table 3**); the components of the dialysate fluids (**Table 4**). Proposed in the Ansari article [45] are multiple and involve the following elements.

Several new PD solutions with low-glucose breakdown products have been introduced, but they are more expensive than conventional solutions containing dextrose and lactate. A recent meta-analysis by Sheng et al. [57] concludes that PD solution with low-glucose breakdown products preserves residual renal function and improves dialysis adequacy without increasing all-cause mortality. Further trials are needed to determine whether this beneficial effect may affect long-term clinical outcomes.

Recommendations on the choice of peritoneal dialysis (PD) fluids in children [58] conclude that the concentration of glucose should be as low as possible in the dialysate fluid. Icodextrin can be applied once a day during prolonged hospitalisation, particularly in children with inadequate ultrafiltration. Infants on PD are at risk of sodium depletion associated with ultrafiltration, while anuric adolescents may experience water and salt overload. The sodium-chloride balance must therefore be closely monitored. In growing children, the calcium balance should be positive, and the calcium in the dialysate should be adjusted according to individual needs.

Amino acid-based PD fluid in children suggests good tolerance. However, the anabolic effect is weak; adequate enteral nutrition is preferable.

Composition of the dialysate fluid
1. Sodium 132–134 (mmol/L)
2. Potassium 0–2 (mmol/L)
3. Calcium 1.25–1.75 (mmol/L)
4. Magnesium0.25–0.75 (mmol/L)
5. Chloride 95–106 (mmol/L)
6. Lactate 35–40 (mmol/L) or HCO3 (34 mmol/L)
7. Glucose 1.5–4.25 (g/dL)
8. pH (Neutral and physiological in newer peritoneal dialysis fluid preparations).

Table 3.
The composition of the dialysate fluide.

Components	Comments
Length of the dialysis session	Length of dialysis session determined by fluid balance, biochemical abnormalities and urine output
Composition of dialysate (% dextrose)	Ultrafiltration rate of 1.5% dextrose and 2.5% dextrose (40 ml/kg dwell) is 50–150 and 200–400 ml/h, respectively. A higher concentration of dextrose solution may be used for initial cycles in children with severe fluid overload.
Exchange volume	Initial fill volume: 10–20 ml/kg; maximum fill volume: 30 ml/kg or 1100 ml/m^2, but <800 ml/m^2 if age < 2 years. The higher the fill volume, the greater the clearance and ultrafiltration.
Exchange time—inflow, dwell, outflow time	Initial exchange time is 1 h—inflow 10 min, dwell 30–40 min, outflow 20 min. Dwell time pf 1–4 h in continuous PD using a flexible catheter. Shorter dwell time for rapid fluid, urea and potassium clearance (e.g. severe hyperkalaemia or pulmonary oedema). If hypernatremia develops, extend the dwell time if feasible or lower glucose concentration in dialysis solution.
Additives to dialysate	Potassium 3–4 mmol/l Heparin 250–1000 U/l
Monitoring	Fluid balance q 4–6 h Serum electrolytes per 6–12 h Blood sugar per 6–12 h (more frequently if using 2.5 or 4.25% dextrose-based dialysis fluid) Blood urea and serum creatinine per 24 h

PD, Peritoneal dialysis.

Table 4.
The components of the dialysate fluids.

In our daily practice in the intensive care unit at the university hospital, the nursing team uses a closed manual system, based on gravity, to deliver the dialysis fluid and drain it from the peritoneal cavity. In neonates, we use burettes to adapt the inflow and outflow of dialysis fluid.

6.4 Regimen of peritoneal dialysis

The different regimes have been described: intermittent peritoneal dialysis (IPD), and modifications to PD have been made recently to improve ultrafiltration, namely continuous equilibration PD, high volume PD, tidal PD, and continuous flow PD [59, 60].

Intermittent peritoneal dialysis (IPD) often used in our hospital for infants, using a rigid catheter. The infusion, contact, and draining times make up 1 cycle of 1 hour. This regime can be carried out manually or using a cycler by prescribing a pre-determined volume of dialysate fluid to drain the peritoneal cavity.

In children, 30 to 40 mL/kg of dialysate, warmed to 37°C, is infused over 10 to 15 minutes, then sucked back into the peritoneal cavity over 30 to 40 minutes, and drained after 10 to 15 minutes. Short exchanges of 1 to 2 L are carried out in sessions lasting 16 to 24 hours, three times a week.

Continuous PD is similar to continuous ambulatory peritoneal dialysis (CAPD), in which manual exchange is performed every 3 to 6 hours depending on patient clearance and fluid elimination.

It requires multiple daily exchanges, either manually or using a cycler. The disadvantage of this regime is that the patient must be hospitalised, and clearance may be insufficient, particularly in hypercatabolic patients, due to a lower dialysate flow rate [35].

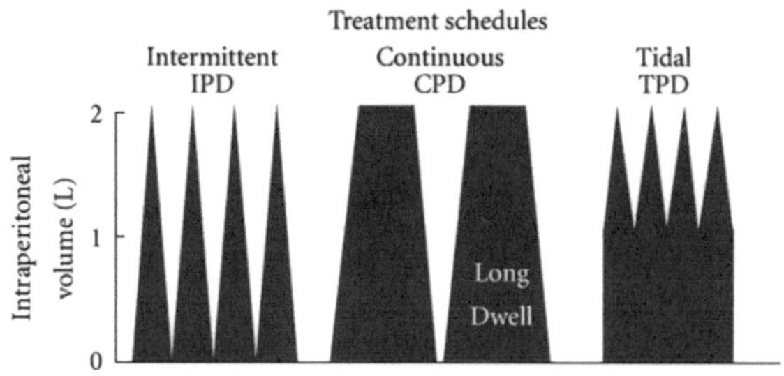

Figure 1.
Basic mechanisms operating in various peritoneal dialysis regimens adapted from Ansari [45].

Tidal peritoneal dialysis (TPD) requires a cycler and is a modality in which only part of the dialysate (25–50% of the infused volume) after a pause is drained during a long session lasting 8 to 10 hours, but optimisation of the clearance of drained solutes is not satisfactory [61, 62].

Basic mechanisms operating in various peritoneal dialysis regimens adapted from Ansari [45] are summarised in **Figure 1**.

6.5 Prescription of peritoneal dialysis

The prescription of PD must take into account the patient's clinical condition, body surface area, and state of hydration in order to achieve better ultrafiltration.

To initiate dialysis, it is recommended that the filling volume be calculated on the basis of body surface area rather than on the basis of the child's weight to avoid the problem of peritoneal membrane hyperpermeability.

It is recommended that the peritoneal cavity be filled with dialysate fluid with a volume of 10–20 ml/kg or 300–600 ml per body surface area in infants until the desired volume is obtained in the order of 30 ml/kg (800 ml per body surface area according to recommendations). There is a gradual increase in volume between d2 and d14 Up to 900 ml/m^2 body surface area for infants and 1400 ml/m^2 in older children.

Increasing the volume of dialysate must be done with caution, because although it improves diffusion and ultrafiltration, it also increases the risk of leakage and therefore of infection, and may create discomfort and thus a compliance defect [63].

In an article, Fischback et al. [64] describe a relationship between intraperitoneal hydrostatic pressure and dialysate volume in children on PD and demonstrate that the relationship between intraperitoneal pressure (IPP) and infused peritoneal volume (IPV) depends on age. In neonates, stable PPI values (3.5 +/− 1.6 cm) were observed for IPVs of 600 to 800 ml/m^2. Mean intraperitoneal pressure values were 8.2 +/− 3.8 cm for a mean peritoneal volume of 990 +/− 160 mL/m^2 body surface area, no significant increase in mean IPP was observed in infants (4.8 +/− 2.6 cm) and children (9.6 +/− 2.1 cm), and the increase in IPP was substantial when IPV increased from 1200 to 1400 mL/m^2 [64].

The dialysis cycle, which may last 60 to 90 minutes, includes a filling time, a pause or contact time of 30 to 40 minutes, and a drainage time.

In the event of threatening hyperkalaemia or a hypercatabolic state, the contact time may be reduced to ensure a high flow rate and therefore effective dialysis, especially in small children.

The duration of contact time in chronic dialysis for children with acute CPP is approximately 3 to 6 hours, which can be shortened to increase the total number of exchanges in order to improve solute clearance.

In acute PD, the duration of dialysis sessions will depend on the doses of dialysis administered, electrolyte and metabolic balance, and the daily kinetics of blood urea and creatinine.

Treatment is monitored on an hourly basis and reports on the amount of fluid recovered during each cycle, the type of dialysate used, its volume, any difficulties encountered, and tolerance. The input and output results and the ionogram enable prescriptions to be adjusted and the effectiveness of PD to be assessed.

Table 4 summarises components of acute peritoneal dialysis prescription adapted by Vasudevan and colleagues [65].

6.6 Complications

Numerous complications are inherent in peritoneal dialysis, and we summarise the main complications associated with this type of APD.

- Infectious complications: Despite improvements in techniques over the last few decades, infectious peritonitis remains one of the most feared complications [66]. Infectious peritonitis may be caused by contamination during handling, infection of the orifice through continuity, bacterial translocation through the digestive wall, or perforation of a hollow organ. The causative organisms are gram-positive and gram-negative bacteria. Peritonitis is suspected when the drainage fluid is cloudy. The diagnosis is confirmed by analysis of the drainage fluid for cell count, culture, and antibiotic sensitivity. Broad-spectrum antibiotic therapy should be initiated as soon as empirically possible to avoid the serious consequences of peritonitis, such as sepsis, and catheter removal.

    - Mechanical complications: Pain on instillation of the liquid or on drainage is a known complication in PD patients, occurring in 13 to 25% of cases [67].

Several factors contribute to this pain: low pH of the dialysate fluid, low temperature, or distension of the tissues around the catheter.

This pain can be minimised by infusing an alkaline PD fluid adding sodium bicarbonate and increasing the temperature of the dialysate while slowing the rate of dialysate infusion [46].

6.7 Intra-abdominal haemorrhage

Mild intra-abdominal haemorrhage is common and may be observed during catheter insertion. Severe intra-abdominal haemorrhage has been reported, particularly with acute semi-rigid catheters.

6.8 Intestinal perforation

Intestinal perforation may occur, particularly with the use of semi-rigid catheters in acute PD. Patients may experience severe abdominal pain, blood-stained peritoneal fluid, intra-abdominal haemorrhage, and (rarely) shock. Treatment consists of stopping treatment for a short period, removing the catheter, administering intravenous antibiotics, and treating the bowel.

Mechanical complications have been reported in several series, including leakage at the catheter insertion site, catheter occlusion, inguinal hernia, catheter malfunction, and fluid leaks [66, 68].

Respiratory complications such as:

- Respiratory distress during infusion of peritoneal fluid in children when the drainage fluid was insufficient, which increases intraperitoneal pressure; recommendations must be taken into consideration when infusing fluid according to the child's size and weight.

- Hydrothorax, generally on the right, is rare and is due to the presence of a congenital diaphragmatic anomaly with subsequent pleuroperitoneal communication, lymphatic drainage, and a pleuroperitoneal pressure gradient. Severe cases may require discontinuation of PD and surgical closure of the septal defect.

Pleurodesis by insufflation of talcum powder or thoracoscopic pleurodesis has been carried out in certain published series [69–71].

6.9 Metabolic complications

Hyperglycaemia can result from a high concentration of glucose in the PD fluid.

- Hypoglycaemia may occur as soon as PD is stopped.

- Hypernatremia: This can be induced by the disproportionate loss of free water in the PD fluid when hypertonic exchanges are frequently used. This is because the aquaporin-1 water channels in the capillaries are activated by the tonicity of the glucose generated by the dialysate. However, if the exchange is of short duration, sodium diffusion can take place early enough, and the patient slowly becomes hypernatremic. Ideally, the duration of the exchange should be corrected for diffusion to occur, or a hypertonic dialysate should be used.

Lactic acidosis is rare, except in patients with end-stage liver failure.

Lactic acidosis can be avoided by the use of peritoneal dialysis fluid containing bicarbonate.

- Hypokalaemia is frequently observed as standard dialysate fluid is at a concentration of 0–2 (mmol/L). Consideration should be given to the empirical addition of potassium to the dialysate solution after 12 hours of continuous PD in order to achieve a concentration of 3–4 mmol/L in the dialysate [42].

Volume changes may occur as a result of the use of hyperosmotic fluid leading to hypovolaemia or ultrafiltration failure leading to hypervolaemia, especially in the event of an episode of acute peritonitis.

This problem of volume imbalance can be resolved by adjusting the dialysis prescription or, in certain situations, necessitating temporary cessation of dialysis.

During episodes of acute peritonitis, hypoalbuminemia may develop due to high protein losses in the dialysate, which may reach 10 to 20 grams per day, requiring protein intake to be increased on a daily basis by infusing albumin.

Table 5 shows the complications associated with peritoneal dialysis and possible suggestions for their management, adapted by Nourse [42].

Initial prescription	Fill volume: 10–20 ml/kg Total cycle: 60–90 min. Fill: 5–10 min; dwell: 30–60 min; drain: 10–20 min Initial glucose concentration: 2.5% Heparin 500 IU/I PD over a full 24-h for 1–3 days
Problem	*Modification to prescription*
Poor ultrafiltration	1. Rule out access issues or peritoneal leak 2. Increase glucose concentration (1.5% → 2.5% → 4.25%) (or 1.36, 2.27 and 3.86% in some areas) 3. Decrease exchange duration by reducing dwell time by +25% (reduce fill and drainage times to a minimum) 4. Increase fill volumes 30–40 ml/kg (800–1100 ml/m^2) 5. Consider CFPD
Hyperkalaemia (emergency treatment required)	1. Reduce dwell time to 15–30 min (reduce fill and drainage times to a minimum) 2. Monitor potassium levels regularly
Serum potassium <4 mmol/l	Add 4 mmol/l of potassium to PD fluid
Difficulty with ventilation/increased intra-abdominal pressure	1. Reduce fill volume incrementally by 5 ml/kg. 2. Position patient in semi-fowlers position (30° head up) 3. Consider measuring intra-abdominal pressure to guide fill volume (either intravesical pressure with a transducer *via* a urinary catheter or directly from the PD catheter with a manometer) 4. Consider CFPD with very low fill volumes
High phosphate	1. Tolerate if not problematic and limited duration expected. If problematic: 2. Increase dwell times to >60 min 3. Increase fill volumes 30–40 ml/kg (800–1100 ml/m^2)
Hypernatraemia secondary to rapid cycling	1. Increase dwell time to >60 min 2. Reduce dialysate glucose concentration, if possible
Hypernatraemia, AKI and requiring dialysis	1. Add hypertonic sodium (3% or 5%) to PD fluid to within 15 mmol of patient's sodium to allow a gradual reduction in the serum sodium
Lactic acidosis AND hepatic dysfunction OR shock OR neonate AND/OR not responding to lactate-based fluids	Use bicarbonate-based PD fluids
Hyperglycaemia >20 mmol/l	1. Reduce glucose concentration in PD fluid if possible and/or increase exchange duration 2. If not working or not possible: Insulin infusion (start 0.05 IU/kg/h) OR 3. Add insulin to PD bags (see text Section 3.1)

Development of new pleural effusion	1. Consider extracorporeal dialysis modality if available 2. Insert chest drain and check fluid for glucose 3. Position patient in semi-fowlers position (30° head up) 4. Reduce volume of PD per cycle 5. Measure volume of fluid coming from chest drain and add to fluid balance

PD: peritoneal dialysis; AKI: acute kidney injury; CFPD: continuous flow peritoneal dialysis.

Table 5.
Complications associated with peritoneal dialysis and possible suggestions for their management.

7. Timing of initiation of peritoneal dialysis

Apart from the severity criteria for AKI requiring an emergency dialysis session, in the paediatric literature there is no optimum time to start a PD session.

Very few studies have evaluated the potential benefits of starting EBRT early.

The paediatric series found in the literature are debatable. Early initiation of renal replacement therapy in paediatric heart surgery is associated with lower mortality.

In a retrospective study of 146 newborn babies and children treated with peritoneal dialysis following cardiac surgery in a referral hospital, the authors noted that mortality was 28.1% at 30 days and 36.3% during follow-up. Early dialysis was associated with a 46.7% reduction in 30-day mortality and a 43.5% reduction in 90-day mortality compared with late dialysis. All other short-term variables were similar. Initiation of peritoneal dialysis on the day of surgery or the first day after surgery was associated with a significant reduction in mortality [72].

Another study conducted by Sanchez-de-Toledo et al. showed that early dialysis reduced mortality after paediatric cardiac surgery, and thus the relationship between RIA and morbidity and mortality after paediatric cardiac surgery. A single-centre retrospective study of children who underwent paediatric cardiac surgery between April 2010 and December 2012 in a tertiary hospital included 480 patients. Of these, 109 (23%) were neonates, and 126 infants and children (26%) developed AKI within the first 72 hours postoperatively. RRT techniques were used in 32 (6.6 %) patients (16 %) neonates and (3.8 %) infants and children; $p < 0.01$, with 78% receiving peritoneal dialysis (PD) and 22% continuous EER (CRRT). Patients treated with PD within the first 24 hours postoperatively had lower mortality than those in whom PD was initiated later [4/16 (25%) vs. 4/9 (44.4%)]. Mortality in patients who received CRRT late was 28.6%; no deaths were reported in patients treated with CRRT within the first 24 hours postoperatively [73].

In a meta-analysis conducted by Karvellas et al. [74], 15 studies (2 randomised, 4 prospective cohorts, and 9 retrospective cohorts) were identified out of 1494 citations. The overall methodological quality was poor. Early treatment of ERA compared with late treatment was associated with a significant improvement in 28-day mortality (odds ratio (OR) 0.45; 95% confidence interval (CI), 0.28 to 0.72). However, the limitations of this meta-analysis revealed significant heterogeneity as patients were stratified into medical and surgical patients. The prospective and retrospective study design and the early time to initiation of dialysis were not well defined.

8. Impact of PD on outcomes in children with AKI

There are limited data on the effect of EER modality on survival in paediatric AKI patients.

A retrospective study by Fleming et al. [38] compared HDF (n = 21) and PD (n = 21) in 42 children following repair of congenital heart defects. They concluded that haemodialfiltration (HDF) was superior to PD in terms of ultrafiltration and better nutritional support but no survival benefit was demonstrated between the modalities.

Bunchman et al. [75] in a retrospective study over 7 years reviewed survival outcomes in 226 paediatric patients receiving various forms of RRT, including PD, IHD, and CRRT.

A total of 106 patients were treated with CRRT, 61 with HDF, and 59 with PD. About 54% of the total population studied survived: 40% in the haemofiltration group. About 49% in the group treated with peritoneal dialysis, and 81% in the group treated with intermittent haemodialysis. Despite the clear superiority of IHD over the other modalities in this study, the authors concluded that haemodynamic instability better predicted greater mortality than the EER modality.

Regarding PD regimen: A prospective study by Gabriel et al. [76] was performed on 30 AKI patients who were assigned to continuous high-dose PD (Kt/V = 0.65 per session) *via* a flexible catheter (Tenckhoff) and to automated PD with a cycler. Fluid removal, pH and metabolic control, protein loss, and patient progress were assessed. Patients received 236 sessions of continuous PD, with standardised values for creatinine clearance and urea Kt/V of 110.6+/−22.5 L/week/1.73 m(2) body surface area and 3.8+/−0.6, respectively. Regarding the outcome of AKI, 23% of patients recovered renal function, 13% remained on dialysis after 30 days of follow-up, and 57% died.

A multicentre cohort study [77] was conducted on patients over 15 years of age admitted to an intensive care unit and diagnosed with acute renal failure. The aim of the study was to determine the effects of renal replacement therapy (RRT) modalities on 30-day mortality and renal recovery in patients with AKI whose main aetiology is sepsis.

Intermittent haemodialysis (IHD), continuous renal replacement therapy (CRRT), peritoneal dialysis (PD), or sustained low-efficiency dialysis (SLED) were the treatment modalities (of the 2844 patients with AKI, 449 cases (8.1%) received CRRT). There were no significant differences in 30-day mortality between patients initially treated with CRRT (52%), PD (51.6%), and SLED (55.6%) compared with those treated with HDI. Renal recovery was similar for each RRT mode.

9. Conclusion

The choice of technique for the treatment of AKI depends on the size of the patient, the availability of vascular access, the integrity of the peritoneal membrane and the abdominal cavity, as well as the clinical experience and expertise of the practitioner.

However, in most developing countries, as is the case in Africa, access to paediatric haemodialysis is difficult, so PD remains the only option available for the treatment of AKI.

PD still has its place in paediatric intensive care, particularly in patients with AKI due to a disease at risk of chronic renal failure.

To limit complications, particularly peritonitis, surgical placement of the catheter and strict compliance with a care and monitoring protocol are recommended.

Training of care teams and close collaboration with paediatric resuscitators and paediatric nephrologists are essential.

Conflict of interest

The authors declare no conflict of interest.

Author details

Djamila Djahida Batouche[1,2,3]*, Djilali Batouche[4], Zakaria-Zoheir Addou[1,2], Dalila Boumendil[2] and Fatima Souhila Bouchama[2]

1 Paediatric Neonatal Intensive Care Unit EHU, Oran, Oran, Algeria

2 Faculty of Medicine Oran 1, Oran, Algeria

3 Research Laboratory LERMER, University Oran 1, Oran, Algeria

4 Clinical Research Multihealth and Pharmacovigilance, Company Freelance, Paris, France

*Address all correspondence to: batouchedjamiladjahida@gmail.com

References

[1] Prandota J. Clinical pharmacology of furosemide in children: A supplement. American Journal of Therapeutics. 2001;**8**(4):275-289. DOI: 10.1097/00045391-200107000-00010

[2] Warady BA, Bunchman T. Dialysis therapy for children with acute renal failure: Survey results. Pediatric Nephrology. 2000;**15**(1-2):11-13. DOI: 10.1007/s004670000420

[3] Flynn JT, Kershaw DB, Smoyer WE, Brophy PD, McBryde KD, Bunchman TE. Peritoneal dialysis for management of pediatric acute renal failure. Peritoneal Dialysis International. 2001;**21**(4):390-394. PMID: 11587403

[4] Goldstein SL, Currier H, Graf CD, Cosio CC, Brewer ED, Sachdeva R. Outcome in children receiving continuous venovenous hemofiltration. Pediatrics. 2001;**107**:1309

[5] Batouche D-D, Kerboua K. Pronostic prognosis-of-acute-renal-failure-in-children-in-intensive-care-unit-a-pilot-study. Current Pediatric Research. 2019;**20**(2):194-119

[6] Akran-Arikan A, Zappitelli M, Loftis LL, Washburn KK, Jefferson LS, Goldstein SL. Modified RIFLE criteria in critically ill children with acute kidney injury. Kidney International. 2007;**71**:1028e35

[7] Mehta RL, Kellum JA, Shah SV, Molitoris BA, Ronco C, Warnock DG, et al. Acute kidney injury network: Report of an initiative to improve outcomes in acute kidney injury. Critical Care. 2007;**11**(2):R31

[8] KDIGO Clinical Practice Guideline for Acute Kidney Injury. Kidney International Supplements. Vol. 2, No. 1. 2012. DOI: 10.1038/kisup.2012.1

[9] Xu X, Nie S, Zhang A, Jianhua M, Liu HP, Xia H, et al. A new criterion for pediatric AKI based on the reference change value of serum creatinine. Journal of the American Society of Nephrology: JASN. 2018;**29**(9):2432-2442. DOI: 10.1681/ASN.2018010090

[10] Sutherland SM, Byrnes JJ, Kothari M, Longhurst CA, Dutta S, Garcia P, et al. AKI in hospitalized children: Comparing the pRIFLE, AKIN, and KDIGO definitions. Clinical Journal of the American Society of Nephrology. 2015;**10**:554-561

[11] Selewski DT, Charlton JR, Jetton JG, Guillet R, Mhanna MJ, Askenazi DJ, et al. Neonatal acute kidney injury. Pediatrics. 2015;**136**(2):e463-e473

[12] Williams DM, Sreedhar SS, Mickell JJ, Chan JC. Acute kidney failure: A pediatric experience over 20 years. Archives of Pediatrics & Adolescent Medicine. 2002;**156**(9):893-900. DOI: 10.1001/archpedi.156.9.893. PMID: 12197796.

[13] Mehta P, Sinha A, Sami A, Hari P, Kalaivani M, Gulati A, et al. Incidence of acute kidney injury in hospitalized children. Indian Pediatrics. 2012;**49**:537-542. DOI: 10.1007/s13312-012-0121-6. Epub 2011 Dec 17. PMID: 22317984

[14] Raina R, Chauvin AM, Bunchman T, Askenazi D, Deep A, Ensley MJ, et al. Treatment of AKI in developing and developed countries: An international survey of pediatric dialysis modalities. PLoS One. 2017;**12**(5):e0178233. DOI: 10.1371/

journal.pone.0178233. PMID: 28557999; PMCID: PMC5448754

[15] Coulthard MG, Vernon B. Managing acute renal failure in very low birthweight infants. Archives of Disease in Childhood. 1995;**73**:F187-F192. DOI: 10.1136/fn.73.3.f187. PMID: 8535880; PMCID: PMC2528481

[16] Rasmussen SK. An overview of pediatric peritoneal dialysis and renal replacement therapy in infants: A review for the general pediatric surgeon. Seminars in Pediatric Surgery. 2022;**31**:151193. Epub 2022 May 29. PMID: 35725048

[17] Diarrassouba G, Adonis-Koffy L, Niamien E, Yaokreh JB, Coulibaly PA. Acute peritoneal dialysis in African pediatric area experience of pediatric nephrology unit of Yopougon university hospital (Abidjan, Côte d'Ivoire). Blood Purification. 2015;**39**:141-144. DOI: 10.1159%2F000368938. Epub 2015 Jan 20. PMID: 25660135

[18] Menaouri M, Batouche D, Elhalimi K, Hadjou F, Lahmer M, Okbani R, et al. Insuffisance rénale aiguë chez le nouveau-né et son pronostic. Néphrologie & Thérapeutique. 2022;**18**(5):454. DOI: 10.1016/j.nephro.2022.07.057

[19] Rippe B. A three-pore model of peritoneal transport. Peritoneal Dialysis International. 1993;**13**(Suppl. 2):35S-38S. PMID: 8399608

[20] Thiongane A, Ndongo AA, Ba ID, Boiro D, Faye PM, Keita Y, et al. Syndrome hémolytique et urémique de l'enfant au Centre Hospitalier Universitaire (CHU) de Dakar: à propos de quatre observations [Hemolytic-uremic syndrome (HUS) in children at the University Hospital Center in Dakar: about four cases]. Pan African Medical Journal. French. 10 Jun 2016;**24**:138. DOI: 10.11604/pamj.2016.24.138.8822. PMID: 27642476; PMCID: PMC5012731

[21] Moritz ML, Del Rio M, Crooke GA, Singer LP. Acute peritoneal dialysis as both cause and treatment of hypernatremia in an infant. Pediatric. Nephrology. 2001;**16**(9):697-700. DOI: 10.1007/s004670100644. PMID: 11511979

[22] Yildiz N, Erguven M, Yildiz M, Ozdogan T, Turhan P. Acute peritoneal dialysis in neonates with acute kidney injury and hypernatremic dehydration. Peritoneal Dialysis International. May-Jun 2013;**33**(3):290-296. DOI: 10.3747/pdi.2011.00211. Epub 2012 Nov 1. PMID: 23123669; PMCID: PMC3649898

[23] Genc G, Bicakci U, Gunaydin M, Tander B, Aygun C, Ozkaya O. Temporary peritoneal dialysis in Newborns and children: A single-center experience over five years. Renal Failure. 2012;**34**(9):1058-1061. DOI: 10.3109/0886022X.2012.715574. Epub 2012 Aug 20. PMID: 22906229

[24] Tomar A, Kumar V, Saha A. Peritoneal dialysis in children with sepsis-associated AKI (SA-AKI): An experience in a low- to middle-income country. Paediatrics and International Child Health. 2021;**41**(2):137-144. DOI: 10.1080/20469047.2021.1874201. Epub 2021 January 17. PMID: 33455545

[25] Basu B, Mahapatra TK, Roy B, Schaefer F. Efficacy and outcomes of continuous peritoneal dialysis versus daily intermittent hemodialysis in pediatric acute kidney injury. Pediatric Nephrology. 2016;**31**(10):1681-1689. DOI: 10.1007/s00467-016-3412-7

[26] Mwaba C, Munsaka S, Bvulani B, Mwakazanga D, Chiluba BC, Fitzwanga K, et al. Malaria is the leading

cause of acute kidney injury among a Zambian paediatric renal service cohort retrospectively evaluated for aetiologies, predictors of the need for dialysis, and outcomes. PLoS One. 2023;**18**(10):e0293037. DOI: 10.1371/journal.pone.0293037. PMID: 37878602; PMCID: PMC10599569

[27] Kwiatkowski DM, Krawczeski CD. Acute kidney injury and fluid overload in infants and children after cardiac surgery. Pediatric Nephrology. 2017;**32**(9):1509-1517. DOI: 10.1007/s00467-017-3643-2. Epub 2017 Mar 30. PMID: 28361230

[28] Li H, Yang S, Jin L, Wang Z, Xie L, Lv J, et al. Peritoneal dialysis treatment in small children with acute kidney injury: Experience in Northwest China. Blood Purification. 2019;**48**(4):315-320. DOI: 10.1159/000502079 [Epub 2019 Jul 29]. PMID: 31357204

[29] McCulloch M, Abugrain K, Mosalakatane T, Coetzee A, Webb K, Scott C. Peritoneal dialysis for treatment of acute kidney injury in a case of paediatric inflammatory multisystem syndrome temporally associated with SARS-CoV-2. Peritoneal Dialysis International. 2020;**40**(5):515-517. DOI: 10.1177/0896860820953716. Epub 2020 Sep 2. PMID: 32875970

[30] Parapiboon W, Ponce D, Cullis B. Acute peritoneal dialysis in COVID-19. Peritoneal Dialysis International. 2020;**40**(4):359-362. DOI: 10.1177/0896860820931235. Epub 2020 Jun 19. PMID: 32552550

[31] Al-Hwiesh AK, Mohammed AM, Elnokeety M, Al-Hwiesh A, Al-Audah N, Esam S, et al. Successfully treating three patients with acute kidney injury secondary to COVID-19 by peritoneal dialysis: Case report and literature review. Peritoneal Dialysis International. 2020;**40**(5):496-498. DOI: 10.1177/0896860820953050. PMID: 32998645

[32] Chen W, Caplin N, El Shamy O, Sharma S, Sourial MY, Ross MJ, et al. NYC-PD Consortium. Use of peritoneal dialysis for acute kidney injury during the COVID-19 pandemic in New York City: A multicenter observational study. Kidney International. 2021;**100**(1):2-5. DOI: 10.1016/j.kint.2021.04.017. Epub 2021 April 28. PMID: 33930411, PMCID: PMC8079266

[33] Golej J, Kitzmueller E, Hermon M, Boigner H, Burda G, Trittenwein G. Low-volume peritoneal dialysis in 116 neonatal and paediatric critical care patients. European Journal of Pediatrics. 2002, 2002;**161**(7):385-389. DOI: 10.1007/s00431-002-0919-7. Epub 2002 May 9. PMID: 12111191

[34] Bunchman TE, Meldrum MK, Meliones JE, Sedman AB, Kershaw DB. Pulmonary function variation in ventilator dependent critically ill infants on peritoneal dialysis. Advances in Peritoneal Dialysis. 1992;**8**:75-78. PMID: 1361858

[35] Chitalia VC, Almeida AF, Rai H, Bapat M, Chitalia KV, Acharya VN, et al. Is peritoneal dialysis adequate for hypercatabolic acute renal failure in developing countries? Kidney International. 2002;**61**(2):747-757. DOI: 10.1046/j.1523-1755.2002.00177.x. PMID: 11849419

[36] Chionh CY, Soni S, Cruz DN, Ronco C. Peritoneal dialysis for acute kidney injury: Techniques and dose. Contributions to Nephrology. 2009;**163**:278-284. DOI: 10.1159/000223811. Epub 2009 Jun 3. PMID: 19494626

[37] Schaefer F, Straube E, Oh J, Mehls O, Mayatepek E. Dialysis in neonates with

inborn errors of metabolism. Nephrology, Dialysis, Transplantation. 1999;**14**:910-918. DOI: 10.1093/ndt/14.4.910. PMID: 10328469

[38] Fleming F, Bohn D, Edwards H, Cox P, Geary D, McCrindle BW, et al. Renal replacement therapy after repair of congenital heart disease in children. A comparison of hemofiltration and peritoneal dialysis. The Journal of Thoracic and Cardiovascular Surgery. 1995;**109**(2):322-331. DOI: 10.1016/S0022-5223(95)70394-2. PMID: 7853885

[39] Krause I, Herman N, Cleper R, Fraser A, Davidovits M. Impact of dialysis type on outcome of acute renal failure in children: A single-center experience. The Israel Medical Association Journal (IMAJ). 2011;**13**(3):153-156

[40] Gabriel DP, Caramori JT, Martim LC, Barretti P, Balbi AL. High volume peritoneal dialysis vs daily hemodialysis: A randomized, controlled trial in patients with acute kidney injury. Kidney International. 2008;**73**(Suppl. 108):S87-S93. DOI: 10.1038/sj.ki.5002608. PMID: 18379555

[41] Cullis B, Al-Hwiesh A, Kilonzo K, McCulloch M, Niang A, Nourse P, et al. ISPD guidelines for peritoneal dialysis in acute kidney injury: 2020 update (adults). Peritoneal Dialysis International. 2021;**41**:15-31. DOI: 10.1177/0896860820970834. Epub 2020 Dec 3. PMID: 33267747

[42] Nourse P, Cullis B, Finkelstein F, et al. ISPD guidelines for peritoneal dialysis in acute kidney injury: 2020 update (paediatrics). Peritoneal Dialysis International. Mar 2021;**41**(2):139-157. DOI: 10.1177/0896860820982120 [Epub 2021 Feb 1]. PMID: 33523772

[43] De Galasso L, Picca S, Guzzo I. Dialysis modalities for the management of pediatric acute kidney injury. Pediatric Nephrology. 2020;**35**:753-765. DOI: 10.1007/s00467-019-04213-x. Epub 2019 Mar 18. PMID: 30887109

[44] Strazdins V, Watson AR, Harvey B. European Pediatric Peritoneal Sialysis Working Group. Renal replacement therapy for acute renal failure in children: European guidelines. Pediatric Nephrology. 2004;**19**(2):199-207. DOI: 10.1007/s00467-003-1342-7. Epub 2003 Dec 18. PMID: 14685840; PMCID: PMC1766478

[45] Ansari N. Peritoneal dialysis in renal replacement therapy for patients with acute kidney injury. International Journal of Nephrology. 2011;**2011**:739794. DOI: 10.4061/2011/739794. PMID: 21716704; PMCID: PMC3118664 [Epub 2011 Jun 8]

[46] Phu NH, Hien TT, Mai NT, Chau TT, Chuong LV, Loc PP. et al. Hemofiltration and peritoneal dialysis in infection associated acute renal failure in Vietnam. The New England Journal of Medicine. 2002;**347**:895-902. DOI: 10.1056/NEJMoa020074. PMID: 12239258

[47] Al-Hwiesh A, Abdul-Rahman I, Finkelstein F, Divino-Filho J, Qutub H, Al-Audah N, et al. Acute Kidney Injury in Critically Ill Patients: A Prospective Randomized Study of Tidal Peritoneal Dialysis Versus Continuous Renal Replacement Therapy. Therapeutic Apheresis and Dialysis. Aug 2018;**22**(4):371-379. DOI: 10.1111/1744-9987.12660. PMID: 29575788 [Epub 2018 Mar 25]

[48] Cullis B, Abdelraheem M, Abrahams G, Balbi A, Cruz DN, Frishberg Y, et al. Peritoneal dialysis for acute kidney injury. Peritoneal Dialysis International. 2014;**34**(5):494-517.

DOI: 10.3747/pdi.2013.00222. PMID: 25074995; PMCID: PMC4114667

[49] McNiece KL, Ellis EE, Drummond-Webb JJ, Fontenot EE, O'Grady CM, Blaszak RT. Adequacy of peritoneal dialysis in children following cardiopulmonary bypass surgery. Pediatric Nephrology. 2005;**20**(7):972-976. DOI: 10.1007/s00467-005-1894-9. Epub 2005 May 5. PMID: 15875216

[50] Ricci Z, Morelli S, Ronco C, Polito A, Stazi GV, Giorni C, et al. Inotropic support and peritoneal dialysis adequacy in neonates after cardiac surgery. Interactive Cardiovascular and Thoracic Surgery. 2008;7(1):116-120. DOI: 10.1510/icvts.2007.165118. Epub 2007 Nov 30. PMID: 18055480

[51] Xing Y, Sheng K, Liu H, Wu S, Wei H, Li R, et al. Acute peritoneal dialysis is an efficient and reliable alternative therapy in preterm neonates with acute kidney injury. Translational Pediatrics. 2021;**10**(4):893-899. DOI: 10.21037/tp-20-469. PMID: 34012838; PMCID: PMC8107877

[52] Chadha V, Warady BA, Blowey DL, Simckes AM, Alon US. Tenckhoff catheters prove superior to cook catheters in pediatric acute peritoneal dialysis. American Journal of Kidney Diseases. 2000;**35**:1111-1116. DOI: 10.1016/s0272-6386(00)70048-5. PMID: 10845825

[53] Daschner M, Gfrorer S, Zachariou Z, Mehls O, Schaefer F. Laparoscopic Tenckhoff catheter implantation in children. Peritoneal Dialysis International. 2002;**22**(1):22-26. PMID: 11929139

[54] Mattioli G, Castagnetti M, Verrina E, Trivelli A, Torre M, Jasonni V, et al. Laparoscopic-assisted peritoneal dialysis catheter implantation in pediatric patients. Urology. 2007;**69**:1185-1189. DOI: 10.1016/j.urology.2006.12.033. PMID: 17572212

[55] David VL, Mussuto E, Stroescu RF, Gafencu M, Boia ES. Peritoneal dialysis catheter placement in children: Initial experience with a "2+1"-port laparoscopic-assisted technique. Medicina. 2023;**59**(5):961. DOI: 10.3390/medicina59050961. PMID: 37241193, PMCID: PMC10223083

[56] Fischbach M, Warady BA. Peritoneal dialysis prescription in children: Bedside principles for optimal practice. Pediatric Nephrology. 2009;**24**(9):1633-1642. Epub 2008 Sep 20. PMID: 18807074, PMCID: PMC2719743

[57] Chen S, Jia J, Guo H, Zhu N. The benefits of peritoneal dialysis (PD) solution with low-glucose degradation product in residual renal function and dialysis adequacy in PD patients: A meta-analysis. Investigación Clínica. Sep 2022;**63**(3):283-303. DOI: 10.54817/ic.v63n3a07

[58] Schmitt CP, Bakkaloglu SA, Klaus G, Schröder C, Fischbach M, European Pediatric Dialysis Working Group. Solutions for peritoneal dialysis in children: Recommendations by the European pediatric dialysis working group. Pediatric Nephrology. 2011;**26**:1137-1147

[59] Kim YH, Resontoc LP. Peritoneal dialysis in critically ill children. In: Deep A, Goldstein SL, editors. Critical Care Nephrology and Renal Replacement Therapy in Children. New York: Springer; 2018. pp. 307-323

[60] Kontesis AKP, George E DM-S, Symvoulidis DA, Komninos Z. Continuous Equilibration Peritoneal Dialysis (CEPD) in Hypercatabolic

Renal FAILURE. Peritoneal Dialysis International. 1983;**3**(4):178-180. DOI: 10.1177/089686088300300404

[61] Balaskas EV, Izatt S, Chu M, Oreopoulos DG. Tidal volume peritoneal dialysis versus intermittent peritoneal dialysis. Advances in Peritoneal Dialysis. 1993;**9**:105-109. PMID: 8105900

[62] Piraino B, Bender F, Bernardini J. A comparison of clearences on tidal peritoneal dialysis and intermittent peritoneal dialysis. Peritoneal Dialysis International. 1994;**14**(2):145-148. PMID: 8043667

[63] Fischbach M, Stefanidis CJ, Watson AR, European Paediatric Peritoneal Dialysis Working Group. Guidelines by an ad hoc European committee on adequacy of the paediatric peritoneal dialysis prescription. Nephrology, Dialysis, Transplantation. 2002;**17**:380-385. DOI: 10.1093/ndt/17.3.380. PMID: 11865081

[64] Fischbach M, Dheu C, Seugé-Dargnies L, Delobbe JF. Adequacy of peritoneal dialysis in children: Consider the membrane for optimal prescription. Peritoneal Dialysis International. 2007;**27**(Suppl. 2):S167-S170. PMID: 17556298

[65] Vasudevan A, Phadke K, Yap HK. Peritoneal dialysis for the management of pediatric patients with acute kidney injury. Pediatric Nephrology. 2017;**32**(7):1145-1156. DOI: 10.1007/s00467-016-3482-6. Epub 2016 October 28. PMID: 27796620

[66] Bakal U, Sarac M, Tartar T, Aydin M, Kara A, Gurgoze MK, et al. Peritoneal dialysis in children infectious and mechanical complications experience of a tertiary hospital in Elazığ, Turkey. Nigerian Journal of Clinical Practice. 2022;**25**(8):1227-1232. DOI: 10.4103/njcp.njcp_1529_21

[67] Ogunc G, Tuncer M, Tekin S, Ersoy F. An unexpected complication in CAPD: Severe abdominal pain. Peritoneal Dialysis International. 2001;**21**:84

[68] Coccia P, Ramírez F, Suárez A, Alconcher L, Balestracci A, Chervo L. Acute peritoneal dialysis, complications and outcomes in 389 children with STEC-HUS: A multicenter experience. Pediatric Nephrology. 2021;**36**(6):1597-1606. DOI: 10.1007/s00467-020-04876-x

[69] Yim AP, Lee TW, Wan IY, Ng C. Images in cardiothoracic surgery. Pleuroperitoneal fistula. The Annals of Thoracic Surgery. Apr 2002;**73**(4):1327. DOI: 10.1016/s0003-4975(01)02743-6. PMID: 11996291

[70] Ramaema DP, Mpikashe P. Pleuroperitoneal leak: An unusual cause of acute shortness of breath in a peritoneal dialysis patient. Case Reports in Radiology. 2014;**2014**:614846. DOI: 10.1155/2014/614846. Epub 2014 Aug 4. PMID: 25165608; PMCID: PMC4137701

[71] Jonny J, Violetta L. Bilateral pleural effusion in continuous ambulatory peritoneal dialysis managed by vats pleurodesis. European Journal of Case Reports in Internal Medicine. 2024;**11**(4):004343. DOI: 10.12890/2024_004343. PMID: 38584902; PMCID: PMC10997387

[72] Bojan M, Gioanni S, Vouhe PR, Journois D, Pouard P. Early initiation of peritoneal dialysis in neonates and infants with acute kidney injury following cardiac surgery is associated with a significant decrease in mortality. Kidney International.

2012;**82**(4):474-481. DOI: 10.1038/ki.2012.172. PMID: 22622499

[73] Sanchez-de-Toledo J, Perez-Ortiz A, Gil L, Baust T, Linés-Palazón M, Perez-Hoyos S, et al. Early initiation of renal replacement therapy in pediatric heart surgery is associated with lower mortality. Pediatric Cardiology. 2016;**37**(4):623-628. DOI: 10.1007/s00246-015-1323-1. PMID: 26687178 Epub 2015 Dec 21

[74] Karvellas CJ, Farhat MR, Sajjad I, Mogensen SS, Leung AA, Ron W, et al. A comparison of early versus late initiation of renal replacement therapy in critically ill patients with acute kidney injury: A systematic review and meta-analysis. Critical Care. 2011;**15**(1):R72. DOI: 10.1186/cc10061

[75] Bunchman TE, McBryde KD, Mottes TE, Gardner JJ, Maxvold NJ, Brophy PD. Pediatric acute renal failure: Outcome by modality and disease. Pediatric Nephrology. 2001;**16**:1067-1071. DOI: 10.1007/s004670100029. PMID: 11793102

[76] Gabriel DP, Nascimento GV, Caramori JT, Martim LC, Barretti P, Balbi AL. High volume peritoneal dialysis for acute renal failure. Peritoneal Dialysis International. May-Jun 2007;**27**(3):277-282. PMID: 17468475

[77] Panaput T, Peerapornratana S, Sirivongrangson P, Kulvichit W, Lumlertgul N, Jonny J. Modalities of renal replacement therapy and clinical outcomes of patients with acute kidney injury in a resource-limited setting: Results from a SEA-AKI study. Journal of Critical Care. 2021;**65**:18-25. DOI: 10.1016/j.jcrc.2021.05.006. PMID: 34058688. Epub 2021 May 23

Chapter 7

Peritoneal Dialysis-Related Complications: A Comprehensive Review

Axler Jean Paul and Abigael Francis

Abstract

Peritoneal dialysis is considered a less invasive, flexible, independent, easy, and financially more accessible technique for patients who require renal replacement therapy. Based on a purification technique using the peritoneum as a filter, it offers the comfort of internal filtration and does not require the complex machinery of traditional hemodialysis. Since its first use many decades ago, progress has been made over the last years to improve the technique and understand the pathophysiological processes regarding the peritoneal membrane. However, peritoneal dialysis remains associated with complications that can be mechanical or more serious and life-threatening, such as peritonitis. Peritoneal dialysis complications are classified as short- or long-term. It is essential to address them, as they are related to increased morbidity, technique failure, transition to hemodialysis, and death but could be preventable. Through this chapter, we will explore these complications, focusing on the most common in terms of incidence and long-term prognosis.

Keywords: complications, peritoneal dialysis, peritonitis, encapsulating, noninfectious, end-stage renal disease

1. Introduction

Peritoneal dialysis is a technique based on the principle of osmosis, which Rene Dutrochet described in the early eighteenth century. It took many years of experimentation, including the installation of a hypertonic solution by Clark et al. at the end of the eighteenth century, to demonstrate the bidirectional permeability of the peritoneum, the evidence described by Babb et al. [1]. However, it was not until advances in cell biology and the electron microscope deciphered the three-pore theory that we mastered transport across the peritoneal membrane, a form of transport known as transcellular transport [1–3]. This technique was essentially experimental. Georges Ganter first used the hypertonic instillation technique on two patients with renal failure. During this period, many tried peritoneal lavage with two catheters, but despite some successful cases, mortality was very high. However, the technique gradually improved until it became the treatment of choice for patients with end-stage renal failure [2–5]. Today, almost 4 million patients with end-stage renal disease use some form of dialysis, 11% of whom use peritoneal dialysis [6].

When considering the potential benefits of peritoneal dialysis, such as improved comfort, the absence of the need for a highly skilled operator, better preservation of residual kidney function, a better alternative for individuals with challenging vascular access, fewer dietary restrictions, and increased social independence for patients at a lower overall cost, it is essential to acknowledge the existence of potential complications [7–12]. In this chapter, we present a thorough review of the most common complications, discussing their frequency, outlook, and possible preventive strategies based on the latest published research. To ensure clarity, we classify the complications into infectious and noninfectious categories.

2. Infectious complications

2.1 Catheter exit-site and tunnel infections

2.1.1 Definitions

Using the catheter during dialysis peritoneally exposes the risk of infection, often presented in two forms that may be concomitant or isolated. These infections are [7, 8]:

- Exit-site infection: A purulent discharge with or without skin erythema at the catheter-epidermis interface. Signs of inflammation (erythema, tenderness, swelling, granuloma, or crust formation) in the absence of discharge are insufficient to diagnose exit-site infection.

- Tunnel infection: Clinical inflammation (erythema, edema, tenderness, induration) with or without ultrasonographic evidence of fluid collection anywhere along the catheter pathway.

2.1.2 Epidemiology and risk factors, causes, and preventable measures

Reported incidence rates vary considerably from country to country, ranging from 0.06 to 0.42 episodes per year [13, 14]. Although the rate of exit-site infections has fallen considerably due to the various preventive measures put in place, it still represents one of the most common complications in peritoneal dialysis patients, with an incidence of 12 per patient-years [8].

The main risk factors are as follows [8].

- Poor competency in exit-site care
- Catheter mobilization
- Catheter pulling-out injury
- Mechanical compression of the catheter by a waist belt
- Swimming
- Presence of pets during exchange
- Compression of the exit site by a peritoneal dialysis catheter bag.

The main germs involved are gram-positive bacteria in 59% of cases, gram-negative bacteria in 23%, fungi in 7%, and 11% in culture-negative cases [8].

2.1.3 Clinical manifestations and diagnosis

Exit-site infections are generally characterized by signs and symptoms like progressive crusting and erythema around the catheter, progressing to the passage of serious then purulent fluid, sometimes accompanied by tenderness and edema. Thus, erythema, edema, induration, and tenderness along the catheter pathway suggest a tunnel infection, which may be complicated by abscess with systemic symptoms such as fever and chills [8].

2.1.4 Prevention and care

Besides the daily dressing, patients with infections should be on antibiotics [7, 8]. Antibiotic ointment should be continued; mupirocin and gentamicin sulfate 0.1% are the most used. The ISPD recommends empirical antibiotic therapy for all peritoneal dialysis patients with exit-site infection, with or without tunnel infection. It generally lasts 3 weeks, and an initial regimen covering *Staphylococcus aureus* is used:

- 1st-generation cephalosporin or penicillinase-resistant penicillin (such as dicloxacillin). In case of allergy to penicillin, clindamycin or trimethoprim/sulfamethoxazole are used.

- Vancomycin should be the first choice in cases of recent infection and colonization with methicillin-resistant *S. aureus* (MRSA).

- Oral ciprofloxacin or intraperitoneal ceftazidime should be added to the initial regimen in cases of previous infection and/or Pseudomonas colonization.

Here are some specific indications that should prompt the removal of the dialysis catheter in case of exit-site and/or tunnel infection:

- Concurrent infection or infection progressing to peritonitis during antibiotic therapy.

- No improvement noted after 3 weeks of adequate antibiotic therapy and/or if the infection is not fully treated after 6 weeks.

- Tunnel or exit-site infection is fungal or mycobacterial in origin.

ISPD recommends that the overall site infection rate be no more than 0.40 episodes per year at risk.

2.2 Peritoneal dialysis-related peritonitis

Peritonitis associated with peritoneal dialysis (PD) is considered the most critical complication, given its mortality. It can lead to, transient loss of ultrafiltration, possible permanent membrane damage, and occasionally death. With any suspicion, it must be evoked, investigated, and treated. The risk of peritonitis secondary to an intra-abdominal and systemic process should also be emphasized, although these cases are relatively rare, accounting for less than 6% [14].

2.2.1 Definition

Peritonitis associated with peritoneal dialysis is defined by the presence of at least two of the following three criteria [7, 14, 15]:

a. Any clinical manifestation suggestive of a diagnosis of peritonitis, such as abdominal pain, signs of peritoneal irritation, and the presence of cloudy peritoneal fluid.

b. On peritoneal fluid analysis, leukocyte counts of >100/micro, or $>0.1 \times 10^9$ (after a dwell time of at least 2 hours), including more than 50% polynuclear leukocytes.

c. Culture-positive dialysis fluids.

Within peritoneal dialysis-related peritonitis, there are several classifications.

- If peritonitis occurs after the dialysis catheter has been inserted but well before the first dialysis session, it is referred to as pre-dialysis peritonitis. Thus, peritonitis associated with dialysis is evoked after the sessions start with the intention to continue with the method [7].

- Culture-negative peritonitis can also occur. It is evoked by the presence of the two above-mentioned clinical criteria.

- Dialysis catheter-related peritonitis is defined as peritonitis co-occurring with an infection of the catheter (tunnel or exit site) or within an interval not exceeding 3 months, with the same organism isolated on analysis of the sample or a sterile sample in the event of prior exposure to antibiotics.

- Peritonitis is recurrent if diagnosed within 4 weeks of completion of therapy of a prior episode incriminating a different organism [1].

- Repeat peritonitis: In this case, peritonitis occurs more than 4 weeks after com pleting treatment for a previous episode with the same microorganism.

- Relapsing peritonitis supposes an episode that occurs within 4 weeks of completion of therapy of a prior episode with the same organism or one sterile episode [1, 7, 16].

- Refractory peritonitis is evoked if, after 5 days of adequate antibiotic therapy, adapted to the results of the peritoneal fluid culture, no improvement is noted, that is, the peritoneal fluid remains cloudy and contains a leukocyte count >100 per 10^9/L. This should automatically lead to removing the dialysis catheter and the recourse to hemodialysis.

2.2.2 Epidemiology

The incidence of peritoneal dialysis-related peritonitis varies widely among countries, ranging from 0.06 episodes/year in Taiwan to 1.66 episodes/year in Israel. However, the incidence rate of PD-related peritonitis has fallen considerably in recent years, from 0.600 episodes/patient-year in 1992 to 0.303 episodes/patient-year in 2019 [17].

2.2.3 Risk factors and preventable measures

Although it still represents a significant challenge and one of the main barriers to using peritoneal dialysis, several studies have demonstrated a significant reduction in infectious complications associated with it over the last 10–20 years, particularly peritonitis [10].

The most related risk factors for peritonitis related to peritoneal dialysis are summarized below:

- PD system contamination: The peritoneal dialysis exchange system can become contaminated if the sterility chain is breached. This contamination may occur either in a closed system (dry contamination) or in an open system (wet contamination), where the exchange catheter is left open for a prolonged period [7].

  Antibiotic therapy is recommended in open system contamination cases to prevent peritonitis. A retrospective study of 548 episodes of dialysis system contamination revealed a peritonitis rate of 3.1% overall; only cases of open system contamination were complicated by peritonitis (5.6%). Given the lack of data on appropriate antibiotic therapy in these circumstances, the ISPD recommends administering 1 g of intraperitoneal Cefazolin [7, 14].
  Adequate training and correct use of dialysis equipment are recommended. In addition to adequate training, patients must be monitored at home to ensure that the recommendations are followed and the protocol understood [14].

- Dialysis catheter-related infection: Infections of the catheter tunnel and exit site represent a major risk factor for peritonitis [14, 18].

  At least four studies have tested administering IV gentamicin, cefazolin, vancomycin, and cefuroxime. This promotes antibiotic prophylaxis before dialysis catheter insertion to reduce the risk of infectious complications [7, 15].

- Invasive procedures (gastroscopy, colonoscopy, hysteroscopy): Some endoscopic procedures, whether digestive or gynecological, may be followed by peritonitis. Studies have shown that the risk of peritonitis in dialysis patients increases following specific endoscopic procedures such as gastroscopy, hysteroscopy, and colonoscopy, especially when not preceded by antibiotic prophylaxis. The rate of occurrence varies from 3.5% to 8.5% for colonoscopy, 1.2% to 3.9% for gastroscopy, and 26.9% to 38.5% for invasive gynecological procedures such as hysteroscopy [7].

- Gastrointestinal disorders (constipation, enteritis): Those disorders have been reported to be associated with peritonitis related to enteric organisms [7, 18].

- *S. aureus* nasal carriage: The nasal cavity represents the main reservoir of *S. aureus*, and *S. aureus* carriage is a risk factor for developing tunnel and exit-site infections in peritoneal dialysis patients. One report demonstrated a 4-fold increase in the risk of exit-site infections in carriers [14].

2.2.4 Clinical manifestations and paraclinical

The symptomatology of peritonitis related to peritoneal dialysis does not differ from that of peritonitis in general. It should be suspected in the presence of any abdominal pain in the population concerned.

Abdominal pain and hazy peritoneal fluid are the symptoms most frequently found in clinical examinations of patients: 79–88% and 84% of cases, respectively. Other signs and symptoms that may appear in the clinical picture are fever (temperature >37.5 C) (29–53%), nausea or vomiting (31–51%), and hypotension (18%). On physical examination, signs of peritoneal irritation, such as abdominal and rebound tenderness, may be noted. Peritoneal fluid sampling followed by analysis remains the test of choice for confirming the diagnosis when performed under appropriate conditions. The leukocyte count in bacterial peritonitis is generally high: >100 cells/mm^3. However, up to 10% of patients may have a lower leukocyte count, even in peritonitis. This may be due to too-short dwell time or a host immune defense that is too weak to elicit an adequate response. Peritoneal fluid cultures are positive in 80–95% of cases, and the organisms most often isolated are gram-positive (e.g., coagulase-negative Staphylococcus species) [15, 16].

2.2.5 Negative culture peritonitis

Culture-negative peritonitis is a clinical peritonitis without any microorganisms identified after sampling and culture [7, 19]. Etiologies can be varied.

1. Infectious: Infectious peritonitis masked by recent antibiotic use, sampling, and culture methods errors, or culture or atypical microorganisms requiring different culture media for an extended period.

2. Noninfectious: Includes peritonitis of chemical or eosinophilic origin.

2.2.6 Management

Antibiotic therapy must be started as soon as peritonitis is suspected, either systemically or intraperitoneally, after appropriate peritoneal fluid sampling for analysis. It must be a broad-spectrum, considering the epidemiology of the environment, and target both gram (+) and gram (−) microorganisms: Cephalosporins 1st generation or vancomycin and Cephalosporins 3rd generation or aminoglycoside respectively [7].

3. Noninfectious complications

Although most of the complications developed by peritoneal dialysis patients are infectious, other non-negligible mechanical and/or metabolic complications can affect this population. A study in a specialized hospital in Bangladesh revealed a 30.9% rate of noninfectious complications in 68 peritoneal dialysis patients. Those complications should be addressed as they can be a cause of technique failure [11, 13, 20].

3.1 Mechanical and/or metabolic complications

3.1.1 Pericatheter leak

Leakage may occur at the catheter insertion site, facilitated by the increased intra-abdominal pressure due to the dialysate infusion into the peritoneal cavity. Methods that may try to prevent this mechanical complication include a break-in period of 2 weeks for patients starting elective PD, performing the therapy lying down, and with a lower infusion volume for the unscheduled beginning of PD. If leakage persists, the catheter must be replaced [6, 9, 15, 16].

3.1.2 Drainage failure/catheter dysfunction

During peritoneal dialysis, the catheter may infuse but not drain (due to constipation, tip migration, or sequestration of the omentum); or the catheter may neither infuse nor drain (due to folds and intramural obstruction). An optimal surgical technique, choice of an appropriate catheter, and adequate postoperative care may help prevent early dysfunction of the catheter. It may require removal and insertion of a new catheter, administration of laxatives for constipation, and omentectomy and/or omentopexy in the case of sequestration [11, 15, 16].

3.1.3 Hernias

The increased abdominal pressure caused by peritoneal dialysis can lead to the formation of hernias, favored by such factors as obesity, recent surgery, dialysate volume, and polycystic kidneys. It is a common complication affecting 12–37% of patients with PD. Surgery may be performed to correct the hernia if the patient has some residual renal function, with resumption of dialysis after 1–2 days [11, 15, 16, 18].

3.1.4 Hydrothorax

Fluid passage through the pleural space may occur through lymphatics or a congenital or acquired diaphragmatic defect. The diagnosis should be made in all non-edematous, dyspneic patients with consistently inadequate ultrafiltration. Pleural fluid analysis will reveal elevated glucose and hypoproteinemia. Treatment consists of lowering intra-abdominal pressure e.g., from continuous ambulatory peritoneal dialysis (CAPD) to Nocturnal automated peritoneal dialysis (APD), discontinuation of peritoneal dialysis for 2–6 weeks, and, as a last resort, pleurodesis, surgical repair or transfer to hemodialysis [15, 16, 18].

3.1.5 Hypokalemia

Hypokalemia is a common complication in patients on continuous PD, with 10–15% requiring potassium supplementation. This may be promoted by the cellular uptake of potassium, prompted by the intraperitoneal glucose load with subsequent insulin release added to intestinal losses. Management may include potassium-sparing diuretics (spironolactone) in chronic cases or intraperitoneal K^+ in acute situations [6, 21].

3.1.6 Other gastrointestinal disorders

PD patients often present gastrointestinal disorders of a gastric and enteric nature. These may include gastrointestinal reflux disease (GERD), dyspepsia, peptic ulcers, delayed gastric emptying, and so on. They are accompanied by signs and symptoms such as nausea, vomiting, fullness, and epigastric discomfort. GERD is favored by increased intraperitoneal pressure, and treatment remains the same as that administered to non-dialysis patients [21].

3.2 Encapsulating peritoneal sclerosis (EPS)

Peritoneal sclerosis remains one of the most critical complications of long-term peritoneal dialysis although very rare. It is characterized by a disproportionate inflammatory response of the peritoneum, leading to fibrosis. It leads to ultrafiltration failure and intestinal obstruction, and the morbidity and mortality associated with this complication are very high [22, 23].

3.2.1 Epidemiology and risk factors

Peritoneal sclerosis is a complication whose annual incidence varies from 0.14% to 2.5%, with a 0.4–8.9% prevalence [23]. The reported incidence rate per 1000 patient-years ranges from 0.7 to 13, a variation explained by limitations in study design and bias detection. The associated mortality rate is around 50% 1 year after diagnosis. Data analysis revealed that survival rates at 1 and 2 years were 67% and 52% in a Dutch registry, respectively.

Several risk factors have been identified that may influence the development of this complication. The most important is the duration of peritoneal dialysis, with a low cumulative incidence rate after 3 years, rising after 5 years.

a. After eight continuous years of peritoneal dialysis, it has been estimated that around 10–20% of patients will develop encapsulating peritoneal sclerosis. A meta-analysis of the risk factors associated with peritoneal dialysis showed that the risk of encapsulated peritoneal sclerosis was higher in patients who had received peritoneal dialysis for a much more extended period (MD: 1.15, 95% CI, 0.68–1.61, P < 0.001) [24].

b. The age at which peritoneal dialysis begins also influences the occurrence of this complication: A lower age at which PD begins is associated with a higher risk of developing encapsulating peritoneal sclerosis.

c. Duration of peritonitis episodes: A meta-analysis of the results of three studies on 1375 patients demonstrated a clear link between peritoneal sclerosis and the duration of peritonitis episodes (MD = 12.66, 95% CI, 3.85–21.47, P = 0.005) [24].

d. The severity and repetition of episodes of peritonitis are also considered predisposing factors for encapsulating peritoneal sclerosis, particularly fungal, *Staphylococcus aureus*, and Pseudomonas infections.

e. Using certain bioincompatible dialysates, others rich in glucose, and the acetate used as a dialysate buffer could represent a risk factor for this complication [25].

f. Data analysis across 6 articles for 9135 patients showed an association between PE and glomerulonephritis. Patients with glomerulonephritis (2413 cases) were at greater risk of developing this complication (OR = 1.42, 95% CI, 1.02–1.97, P = 0.04) [24].

g. Certain drugs, such as beta blockers and calcineurin inhibitors, may also play a predisposing role in the development of peritoneal sclerosis [24].

3.2.2 Diagnosis and clinical manifestations

Encapsulated peritoneal sclerosis is a complication diagnosed primarily through clinical assessment and can be confirmed using imaging and exploratory laparotomy. The most common symptoms include malnutrition (75% with an average body mass index (BMI) of 17.7 kg/m^2), abdominal pain (86%), abdominal distension (82%), and nausea and vomiting (54%). Although the condition generally develops over time, a review of the literature revealed that 29% of patients presented with acute surgical abdomen symptoms such as intestinal obstruction, ischemia, and/or perforation [11, 21].

Early clinical manifestations are nonspecific, and physical examination is often inconclusive. However, some patients may be present with blood-tinged dialysate or ascites. It is only in the later stages that signs of intermittent obstruction (severe cramping, abdominal pain, constipation, and vomiting) appear, and palpation at this stage may reveal an abdominal mass [24].

While not considered the gold standard for diagnosing peritoneal sclerosis, a computed tomography (CT) scan is still the most effective study method. Magnetic resonance imaging (MRI) can also reveal similar findings, providing the added benefit of avoiding exposure to ionizing radiation and offering better visualization of bowel encasement and peritoneal thickening [11, 21, 24, 25].

3.2.3 Prevention and management

The leading risk factor for peritoneal sclerosis is the duration of peritoneal dialysis. Strategies to reduce the risk include temporarily stopping dialysis, using biocompatible dialysates, and reducing the use of glucose-rich dialysates. Encapsulating peritoneal sclerosis management may involve switching to hemodialysis and drug therapy with Tamoxifen and Prednisone. Retrospective analyses have shown a reduction in mortality with Tamoxifen use [11, 18, 21, 24–26].

4. Conclusions

Although peritoneal dialysis is the method of choice for patients requiring renal replacement therapy, mainly because of its financial advantages over hemodialysis, it is not without consequences. It can be accompanied by complications of an infectious nature, such as peritonitis and dialysis catheter-related infections, as well as non-infectious ones, ranging from peritoneal sclerosis to disorders of mechanical origin (peri catheter leak, catheter dysfunction), metabolic (hypokalemia) and miscellaneous (hernias, hydrothorax, gastrointestinal disorders). These complications, especially infectious ones, need to be addressed quickly and appropriately because of the high mortality and morbidity associated with them. The prevention of complications is also an important aspect of the overall management of PD patients, making it essential for all personnel involved, including the patient, to be appropriately trained and to follow guidelines regarding the necessary good practices.

Acknowledgements

The authors acknowledge the use of Grammarly, Inc. software for language polishing of the manuscript.

Conflict of interest

The authors declare no conflict of interest.

Author details

Axler Jean Paul* and Abigael Francis
State University of Haiti, Port-au-Prince, Haiti

*Address all correspondence to: jeanpaulaxler@hotmail.com

References

[1] Babb AL, Johansen PJ, Strand MJ, Tenckhoff H, Scribner BH. Bi-directional permeability of the human peritoneum to middle molecules. Proceedings of the European Dialysis and Transplant Association. 1973;**10**:247-262

[2] Misra M, Phadke GM. Historical milestones in peritoneal dialysis. Contributions to Nephrology. 2019;**197**:1-8

[3] Oreopoulos DG, Thodis E. The history of peritoneal dialysis: Early years at Toronto Western Hospital. Dialysis and Transplantation. 2010;**39**:338-343

[4] Douglas J. Drukker, Parsons and Maher: Replacement of Renal Function by Dialysis 4th Edition. The Ulster Medical Journal. 1997;**66**(1):69. Available from: https://www.ncbi.nlm.nih.gov/pmc/articles/PMC2448713/

[5] Teschner M, Heidland A, Klassen A, Sebekova K, Bahner U. Georg Ganter—A pioneer of peritoneal dialysis and his tragic academic demise at the hand of the Nazi regime. Journal of Nephrology. 2004;**17**(3):457-460

[6] Teitelbaum I. Peritoneal dialysis. New England Journal of Medicine. 2021;**385**(19):1786-1795. Available from: http://www.nejm.org/doi/10.1056/NEJMra2100152

[7] Chow KM, Li PKT, Cho Y, Abu-Alfa A, Bavanandan S, Brown EA, et al. ISPD catheter-related infection recommendations: 2023 update. Peritoneal Dialysis International. 2023;**43**(3):201-219

[8] Nessim SJ. Peritoneal Catheter Exit Site and Tunnel Infections. In: Nissenson AR, Fine RN, Mehrotra R, Zaritsky J, editors. Handbook of Dialysis Therapy. 6th ed. Elsevier; 2023. pp. 268-271. DOI: 10.1016/B978-0-323-79135-9.00026-4. ISBN 9780323791359. Available from: https://www.sciencedirect.com/science/article/pii/B9780323791359000264

[9] Choudhary G, Manapragada PP, Wallace E, Bhambhvani P. Utility of scintigraphy in the assessment of noninfectious complications of peritoneal dialysis. Journal of Nuclear Medicine Technology. 2019;**47**(2):163-168

[10] Mehrotra R, Devuyst O, Davies SJ, Johnson DW. The current state of peritoneal dialysis. Journal of the American Society of Nephrology. 2016;**27**(11):3238-3252

[11] Mihalache O, Doran H, Mustățea P, Bobircă F, Georgescu D, Bîrligea A, et al. Surgical complications of peritoneal dialysis. Chirurgia (Romania). 2018;**113**(5):611-624

[12] Shrestha BM. Peritoneal dialysis or hemodialysis for kidney failure? Journal of Nepal Medical Association. 2018;**56**(210):556-557

[13] Ben, Salem M, Ayed A, Taieb SK, Handous I, Ben Saleh M, Hamouda M, et al. Peritoneal dialysis in Tunisia: Complications, technique and patient's survival (twenty-seven years of experience in a single center). Pan African Medical Journal. 2021;**39**(179):1-13. DOI: 10.11604/pamj.2021.39.179.29354

[14] Kerschbaum J, König P, Rudnicki M. Risk factors associated with peritoneal-dialysis-related peritonitis. International Journal of Nephrology. 2012;**2012**:11.

Available from: https://pmc.ncbi.nlm.nih.gov/articles/PMC3539329/

[15] Szeto CC, Li PKT. Peritoneal dialysis–associated peritonitis. Clinical Journal of the American Society of Nephrology. 2019;**14**:1100-1105

[16] Andreoli MCC, Totoli C. Peritoneal dialysis. Revista da Associação Médica Brasileira. 2020;**66**:37-44

[17] Marshall MR. A systematic review of peritoneal dialysis-related peritonitis rates over time from national or regional population-based registries and databases. Peritoneal Dialysis International. 2022;**42**:39-47

[18] Khan SF. Updates on infectious and other complications in peritoneal dialysis: Core curriculum 2023. American Journal of Kidney Diseases. 2023;**82**:481-490

[19] Tanratananon D, Deekae S, Raksasuk S, Srithongkul T. Evaluation of different methods to improve culture-negative peritoneal dialysis-related peritonitis: A single-center study. Annals of Medicine and Surgery. 2021;**63**:102139. Available from: https://pmc.ncbi.nlm.nih.gov/pmc/articles/PMC7900635/

[20] Bakal U, Sarac M, Tartar T, Aydin M, Kara A, Gurgoze MK, et al. Peritoneal dialysis in children: Infectious and mechanical complications: Experience of a tertiary hospital in Elaziğ, Turkey. Nigerian Journal of Clinical Practice. 2022;**25**(8):1227-1232

[21] Chan R, Walker RJ, Samaranayaka A, Schollum JBW. Long-term impact of early non-infectious complications at the initiation of peritoneal dialysis. Peritoneal Dialysis International. 2023;**43**(1):53-63

[22] Danford CJ, Lin SC, Smith MP, Wolf JL. Encapsulating peritoneal sclerosis. World Journal of Gastroenterology. 2018;**24**:3101-3111

[23] Johnson DW, Cho Y, Livingston BER, Hawley CM, McDonald SP, Brown FG, et al. Encapsulating peritoneal sclerosis: Incidence, predictors, and outcomes. Kidney International. 2010;**77**(10):904-912

[24] Li D, Li Y, Zeng H, Wu Y. Risk factors for Encapsulating Peritoneal Sclerosis in patients undergoing peritoneal dialysis: A meta-analysis. PLoS ONE. 2022;**17**(3)

[25] Hamada C, Tomino Y. Recent understanding of peritoneal pathology in peritoneal dialysis patients in Japan. Blood Purification. 2021;**50**:719-728

[26] Nakayama M, Miyazaki M, Honda K, Kasai K, Tomo T, Nakamoto H, et al. Encapsulating peritoneal sclerosis in the era of a multi-disciplinary approach based on biocompatible solutions: The next-PD study. Peritoneal Dialysis International. 2014;**34**(7):766-774. Available from: www.PDIConnect.com

Chapter 8

Caregiver Burnout and Risk of Peritonitis

Dulce Paola Grajales-García, Jesús Iván Lara-Prado, José Alfredo Feria-Ramírez, Fabiola Pazos-Pérez, Carlos Enrique Mendez-Landa, Yessica Lopez Cabrera, Gustavo Adolfo Bautista Carbajal, Nydia Karen Cruz Escutia, Karla Castillo Carpinteyro and Alejandro Treviño-Becerra

Abstract

Peritonitis is a preventable risk associated with peritoneal dialysis technique. Currently, the elderly population largely bears the burden of CKD, especially in developing countries, where most patients who start dialysis are over 65 years of age and may experience functional decline that demands support from caregivers. In providing assistance, caregivers may experience negative physical and psychological impacts on their quality of life, such as anxiety, depression and burnout syndrome that may lead to peritonitis when caregivers disregard proper technique. Caregiver burnout syndrome is not currently considered a risk factor for peritonitis, therefore we aimed to review the existing literature on this topic and evaluate its frequency among caregivers of patients on maintenance peritoneal dialysis and its possible association with peritonitis.

Keywords: caregiver burnout, peritoneal dialysis, peritonitis risk factors, peritoneal dialysis training, kidney dyad

1. Introduction

The burdens of dialysis disproportionately affect the elderly population and may be associated with functional decline [1], thereby turning some patients dependent on caregivers. In developing countries where long-term care facilities are scarce in the public health system, the role of caregiver is frequently adopted by a patient's relative. This has been termed informal caregiving, as opposed to care received from trained health personnel [2].

The relatively new concept of "caregiving burden" appeared in the 80s and it encompasses the psychological, physical and social impacts on people who care for patients with chronic and debilitating diseases. Informal caregiving has been recently implicated as a risk factor for burnout syndrome [3].

 IntechOpen

Burnout syndrome refers to the psychosocial impact associated with high-stress occupations, which extend to informal caregiving. People who care for patients with chronic diseases frequently experience stress in fulfilling the duties of care in addition to their roles in family, workplace or other social environments [4]. In time, caregivers may gradually place the duties of long-term caring above all other activities, including self-care.

Burnout may be explained, at least, through three dimensions in the caregiving context [2]:

1. *Emotional exhaustion*. Caregivers feel "overloaded" or "drained," and feel they are no longer able to carry on their role as caregivers. When caring.

2. *Depersonalization*. The relationship with the patients becomes detached; in extreme cases, treating the patient as something, instead of someone (termed reification).

3. *Personal accomplishment*. Helping a person who needs care may be a source of meaning and fulfillment. People with burnout may feel that caring has "lost its meaning" or "don't know why" they do it.

Caregiver burnout has a negative social impact especially when the informal caregivers sacrifice their formal job and/or reduce their social interactions with family and friends. These adaptations frequently fail to compensate for the increased stress and eventually lead to physical and mental health issues [5, 6]. In addition to this three-dimensional model, other features that are associated with burnout syndrome include emotional support, coping mechanisms and resilience and adjustment of identity [7]. Attending properly to these factors may even prove beneficial in some cases.

1.1 Epidemiology of caregiver burnout in the setting of CKD

Features of burnout syndrome have been strongly associated with caring for CKD patients, and recent studies have shown a frequency above 50% [8, 9], which may be even higher than that of caregiving in chronic neurological diseases. Dialysis requires major lifestyle adaptations for the patient and their families, and is frequently a long-term treatment, which accounts for the strong association with burnout. Although both dialysis modalities (hemodialysis and peritoneal dialysis) have been implicated, most developing countries do not have home hemodialysis programs, therefore, peritoneal dialysis may pose a greater burden on the caregivers.

1.2 Risk factors for caregiver burnout

Table 1 presents some factors that have been proposed as risk factors for caregiver burnout, which may be attributed to the patient or the caregiver [10–12].

In a systematic review including 38 studies by Alshammarani et al. [13] several factors were identified in relation to burnout syndrome, such as ethnicity, employment, income and religion/spirituality. Besides, they identified other factors related to underlying disease, the environments and situations such as tobacco and alcohol use, as well as level of physical exertion.

Factors from the patient	Factors from the caregiver
Functional status	Age < 70 years
Cognitive status	Female sex
Psychiatric symptoms	Living in the same house as the patient
Behavioral issues	Spousal relationship
Years on dialysis	Sole caregiver
	Educational level

Table 1.
Proposed risk factors for caregiver burnout [10–12].

1.3 Caring for people with CKD: The kidney dyads

The relationship between a person living with CKD and their caregiver can be studied as a dyad [14]. Most frequently, it is a family member who does not receive financial compensation for being the caregiver. In Mexico, CKD patients who begin dialysis are usually over 65 years old and their caregivers are frequently female, often a daughter or spouse, mostly under the age of 55 years [15].

In time, the negative impact of caregiver burnout may extend to the patient on dialysis if the caregiver disregards the PD technique, especially in the setting of functionally impaired patients, who cannot perform the technique on their own. Among dialysis modalities, a study in 180 Mexican patients on peritoneal dialysis showed that continuous ambulatory modality (CAPD) showed higher levels of caregiver burnout, compared to automated PD. This particular group also presented a higher mortality measured one year after the start of dialysis [11].

The healthcare team should consider the various activities and duties of the caregiver in order to identify and treat them properly. Several areas have been identified [16].

- *Domestic duties*. Grocery shopping, preparing meals and house cleaning.
- *Everyday mobility*. Providing aid for personal hygiene, feeding and mobilizing the patient.
- *Healthcare follow up*. Ensuring dialysis technique, treatment compliance and being able to identify the need for urgent medical evaluation.
- *Emotional and social duties*. Providing company, leisure time and conflict resolution.
- *Financial and legal duties*. Including healthcare insurance, advanced care planning and end-of-life care.
- *Dialysis-related*. Technique training and retraining, hand hygiene, prescription, intraperitoneal drug use, and care of the exit site [17].

Ensuring patient compliance includes bearing in mind the dietary restrictions as well as maintaining the proper dialysis technique, which requires longer dedication in

CAPD than in APD patients. Given that CKD is a terminal illness, when the patients invariably reach the end of life, the caregiver frequently accompanies the patient throughout this last stage.

1.4 Identifying caregiver burnout

The negative aspects of the long-term experience of caring may manifest as forms of anxiety or anguish, feelings of fatigued and energy-depleted, deterioration of family relationships, social isolation, excess medication use, and sleep cycle disturbances, with depression-like symptoms. If neglected, by the caregiver or the healthcare personnel, their detrimental effects on health extend beyond the caregiver and negatively affect the patient. Eventually, health systems around the globe will begin experiencing greater workloads and increased costs for attending chronic diseases [18].

Several instruments have been developed to evaluate the symptom burden associated with caregiver burnout **(Table 2)**, with attention to health and quality of life, emotional state, depression, satisfaction with life, family stress, relationship stress, sleep pattern, and sexual health. Specifically, some of them address the subjective experience unique to caring for a family member with a terminal illness.

Escala	Source	Description	Domain or factors	Language
Zarit Burden Interview (ZBI)	Zarit et al. [20]	Subjective	Burdens related to health, psychological well-being, finances, social life and relationship with patient.	English, Spanish, Hebrew, Japanese, Turkish, French, Swedish and Chinese.
Caregiving Burden Scale (CBS)	Gerritsen [21]	Subjective	Burdens related to health, psychological well-being, finances, social life and relationship with patient.	English, Spanish, Japanese, French, Swedish and Chinese.
Caregiving Strain Index (CSI)	Robinsosn [22]	Subjective	Burdens related to employment, financial, physical, social, and time constraints	English
Caregiving Reaction Assessment (CBS)	Given et al. [23]	Subjective	Burdens related to self-esteem, lack of family support, impact on finances, schedule and impact of health	English, Japanese, Thai, Dutch and Korean.
SF-36	Ware et al. [24]	multidimensional	Burdens related to physiological functioning, bodily pain, general health, vitality, social functioning and mental health.	English, Spanish, Japanese, Turkish, French, Swedish and Chinese.
Beck's Depression Inventory (BDI)	Beck et al. [25]	Subjective	Scale was developed as a quantitative measure of depression	English, Spanish, Hebrew, Japanese, Turkish, French, Swedish and Chinese.

Table 2.
Caregiver measurement Instruments [19].

Gilbertson et al. performed a systematic review with 61 high-quality studies, however, they found over 70 different scales were employed [19], They analyzed data on 5367 caregivers of people with chronic dialysis and found that the most frequently used instruments were SF-36, ZBI, CES-D and BDI; due to heterogeneity in the data recollection, comparisons between groups was not possible.

Future studies will be required to standardize the evaluation of burnout syndrome among chronic dialysis caregivers, and importantly, they require cultural adaptation that understands the nuances in cultural significance of the act of caring [26].

Zarit test is one of the most frequently used instruments. Developed in 1980 by Zarit, Reever and Bach-Peterson, it aims to evaluate the caregiving experience and has been translated to and validated in several languages. It consists of 22 items with Likert.type responses, its results vary among the population studied. The Spanish translation has been validated on three categories of burnout: no burnout, mild and moderate–severe [27].

Compared to the general population, quality of life among informal caregivers is lower and similar to the quality of life reported by the very patients with chronic diseases [19].

More recently, Shankar et al. proposed a protocol for systematic evaluation and application of the many tools mentioned before, aiming to select them appropriately to the context of the caregiver [28]. It is necessary that research focuses on longitudinal follow up to better understand the effects of caregiving, considering the dynamic relationship and evolving challenges.

1.5 The impact of caregiver burnout on patients with dialysis

The well-being of caregivers has a direct effect on the healthcare of patients, thus ensuring maximal benefits. This association can be prejudicial, as well. Irianda et al. [11] studied 180 dyads of patients on peritoneal dialysis, and observed that caregiver burnout was associated with an increased frequency of patient hospitalizations, some of which were due to peritonitis (17%), heart failure, surgical procedures and gastrointestinal bleeding. Of the patients admitted with peritonitis, 42% presented caregiver burnout. The most distressing finding in their study was that patients with both a high burden of disease and caregiver burnout had the highest mortality at 12 months.

1.6 Patient and caregiver perspectives on burnout in peritoneal dialysis

It is well known that peritoneal dialysis offers patients a higher degree of autonomy and they have been shown to feel better control over their disease course. However, the dialysis routine can, eventually, overcome the benefits, with many patients disregarding PD or opting for in-center dialysis.

Besides, burnout in the dyad may contribute to low acceptance of PD and be a major contributing factor for dialysis survival. Therefore, many developing countries which rely heavily on PD for most patients with ESKD need to address these issues if they want to increase PD acceptance.

A focus group study with 81 patients and 45 caregivers in Australia, Hong Kong and the USA identified two major themes that contribute to burnout [29].

- The responsibilities are never-ending and undeniable. A feeling of loneliness. “I can’t take it any longer,” “the same routine over and over, it is dialysis or death.”

Caregiving trajectories	Occasional visiting	Daily life activities	Expansion on daily life activities	Long term care facilities	Death
Caregiver tasks	Accompanying medical appointments Monitor and check prescriptions and communication with health professionals	Monitors symptoms and medication Finances and household management Emotional support	Observes changes in behavior, personal hygiene, insurance paperwork	Advance care planning Emotional support	Funeral arrangements Financial issues and insurance paperwork
Effects	Anxiety	Anxiety, anguish	Psychiatric comorbidities	The burden, psychiatric morbidity and stress continue	Recovery: relief and grief Depression

Table 3.
Effects on the caregiver [16].

- Adapting and becoming resilient against burnout requires establishing a "new routine," you accept it and move on (**Table 3**).

2. How to identify peritoneal dialysis-associated peritonitis

Peritonitis should be diagnosed when at least two of the following are present [30]:

1. clinical features consistent with peritonitis, that is, abdominal pain and/or cloudy dialysis effluent;

2. dialysis effluent white cell count >100/μL or > 0.1 × 109/L (after a dwell time of at least 2 h), with >50% polymorphonuclear leukocytes.

3. positive dialysis effluent culture.

2.1 Peritoneal dialysis-associated peritonitis: Impact and prevention

Peritoneal dialysis-associated peritonitis remains the main cause of PD failure. The role of caregiver is only marginally considered as a risk factor by international and national guidelines [30]. A change of caregiver is acknowledged as an indication for PD retraining. Sepsis and peritonitis are the main indications for switching to hemodialysis, and therefore, increase long-term health expenditures [31].

The impact of peritonitis on mortality remains controversial, mainly due to the following concerns:

a. A consensus on the definition of peritonitis-related mortality was achieved in 2022, thereby defined as death occurring within 30 days of the start of peritonitis or during the hospital stay for that cause [30].

b. Indirect long-term effects induced by peritonitis, such as inflammation, malnutrition and functional changes in membrane transport [32–34].

c. Peritonitis is a time-dependent variable which is rarely adjusted for in statistical anaylsis [35].

d. Severe or persistent peritonitis may be associated with intestinal obstruction, perforation and sepsis, which may also be reported as causes of death.

e. Patients with peritonitis are prone to other infectious disease sharing common pathophysiology.

f. Long-term dialysis has been associated with higher alkaline phosphatase as a marker of high-turnover bone disease, which could be an independent risk factor for adverse outcomes in PD [36].

A retrospective cohort of 1321 patients on PD showed that peritonitis is an independent risk factor for all-cause and cardiovascular mortality, after adjusting for age, sex, diabetes, cardiovascular disease, residual kidney function, hemoglobin, phosphorus and albumin [aHR = 1.95, 95% CI 1.45–2.60, $p < 0.001$] [35].

Prevention of peritonitis is endorsed by international guidelines [30], including the following:

- Requesting direct and prompt assessment by the dialysis team if contamination is suspected.

- Administer prophylactic antibiotics after wet contamination of PD connection system. No standard regimen for such antibiotics have been established, and must guide on local antibiotic resistance.

- Antibiotic prophylaxis before invasive routine procedures such as colonoscopy and gynecologic procedures.

- PD exchange technique and knowledge be regularly reassessed and updated, with an emphasis on direct inspection of practice of PD technique.

- Take extra precautions to prevent peritonitis if patients have household pets.

- Avoidance and treatment of hypokalemia may reduce the risk of peritonitis.

In the long-term, efforts to prevent peritonitis and sustain the long-term well-being of the kidney dyads can also have a beneficial impact on public health systems.

2.2 Impact of peritonitis on caregivers

There is scarce research of the consequences of a peritonitis event on the caregiver, sometimes they may express a feeling of guilt, considering that inadequate technique failure drives most of the episodes of peritonitis in ambulatory patients, and perceive the functional deterioration of the patient. These events may eventually precipitate depression requiring medical intervention [37].

2.3 Caregiver burnout and treatment abandonment

Recently, caregiver burnout has been proposed as an important reason behind the decision to withdraw dialysis. Zhang et al. described the most frequent non-medical factors behind withdrawal, mentioning an absence of caregiver, loss of trust in PD and caregiver burnout [31].

Transfer to HD could be a contributing risk factor to mortality. Burn out may be severe enough to require a transfer to HD, despite other indications [38].

3. Professional assisted PD

This strategy is the first choice in developed countries such as the USA, Canada and France, and requires a formal paid caregiver, who performs PD technique. Such personnel may be trained nurses or related health staff who have been properly trained on peritoneal dialysis. The cost of such programs vary from 950 USdollars per day (11,000 USD/year), and is the main barrier that prevents its implementation in developing world [39].

Certain conditions associated with aging may present barriers to caring for oneself and performing PD technique properly, such conditions include sarcopenia, limited hand mobility and fine motor control, visual and auditory impairment, and limited cognitive and learning abilities. A few studies have aimed to evaluate if assistance in home PD increases uptake. Oliver et al. [40] concluded that each of the barriers mentioned above reduces home PD uptake by 26% ($p = 0.02$) and the availability of assistance for home PD increased the likelihood patients would be considered eligible for PD by the multi-disciplinary team There were no statistically significant differences in the choice by the patient whether they were eligible and in PD as a chronic modality between the groups.

Hospitalizations, length of stay, change of modality and death were not different between assisted PD and traditional modalities.

To our knowledge, there are no currently published studies that evaluate PD complications (peritonitis) in the settings of formal vs. informal care; however, a few studies have evaluated the following situations:

- Quality of life and psychosocial effects on the caregiver in assisted PD compared to self-care PD. No statistically significant differences have been found through SF-12,KDQOL-SF, HADS and Zarit test [41].

- Quality of life between PD and HD. No significative differences have been found on caregiver burnout [42].

- Some studies have found a slightly higher frequency of burnout in informal caregivers vs., formal caregivers in HD patients [43].

4. Interventions for preserving caregiver well-being

A growing body of research is now focusing on preserving the well-being of the patient and their caregivers in the long run. So far, there is low-quality evidence to support protocols and psychological support systems of caregivers in the context of CKD and dialysis, such as:

- Caregiver empowerment programs. Group sessions by health personnel (nephrologist, nurse specialist, psychology/psychiatry specialist) focusing on health education and patient-family relationship [44].
- Psychosocial and educational interventions, by individual or group sessions (patient, caregiver and social workers) [45].
- Family-based training, practical workshop, group feedback and techniques for stress management.
- Caregiver-education program. Focusing on the caregivers, sessions are carried in the absence of the patient.
- Load sharing: short-term changes with support from other informal caregivers.
- Flexibility in the dialysis prescription, guidance on schedule modifications in event of emergency.

5. Conclusions

- Caregiver stress and caregiver burnout are common and usually go unnoticed, which can lead to adverse health outcomes for caregivers if not detected and managed in a timely manner.
- Effects of caregiver burnout on the long-term dialysis patient have not been well studied. However, small studies have shown that it can have an effect not only on the cariveger's health but also on the patient's health, even being considered a risk factor for the development of peritonitis.
- There is a need to standardize a validated clinical tool for assessment of caregiver burden in this area.
- Development of optimal information programs on the education and adequate support of family caregivers of dialysis patients should be promoted.

Acknowledgements

Includes funding.

Conflict of interest

The authors declare no conflict of interest.

Author details

Dulce Paola Grajales-García[1*], Jesús Iván Lara-Prado[2], José Alfredo Feria-Ramírez[3], Fabiola Pazos-Pérez[3], Carlos Enrique Mendez-Landa[4], Yessica Lopez Cabrera[3], Gustavo Adolfo Bautista Carbajal[5], Nydia Karen Cruz Escutia[1], Karla Castillo Carpinteyro[6] and Alejandro Treviño-Becerra[7]

1 Regional Hospital No. 1, Mexican Social Security Institute, Mexico City, Mexico

2 General Hospital No. 29, Mexican Social Security Institute, Mexico City, Mexico

3 Specialties Hospital, Mexican Social Security Institute, Mexico City, Mexico

4 General Hospital No. 48, Mexican Social Security Institute, Mexico City, Mexico

5 General Hospital No. 8, Mexican Social Security Institute, Mexico City, Mexico

6 General Hospital No. 27, Mexican Social Security Institute, Mexico City, Mexico

7 National Academy of Medicine, Mexico City, Mexico

*Address all correspondence to: dgrajalesgarcia@gmail.com

References

[1] Kurella-Tamura M, Covinsky KE, Chertow GM, Yaffe K, Landefeld CS, McCulloch CE. Functional status of elderly adults before and after initiation of dialysis. The New England Journal of Medicine. 2009;**361**(16):1539-1547. DOI: 10.1056/nejmoa0904655

[2] Gérain P, Zech E. Informal caregiver burnout? Development of a theoretical framework to understand the impact of caregiving. Frontiers in Psychology. 2019;**10**:1748. DOI: 10.3389/fpsyg.2019.01748

[3] Navaratnarajah A, Clemenger M, McGrory J, Hisole N, Chelapurath T, Corbett RW, et al. Flexibility in peritoneal dialysis prescription: Impact on technique survival. Peritoneal Dialysis International. 2021;**41**(1):49-56

[4] Rohani H, Eslami A, Jafari T, Raei M. The factors affecting the burden of care of informal caregivers of the elderly in Tehran. Kermanshah University of Medical Sciences. 2014;**18**(12):726-736

[5] Kuzuya M, Enoki H, Hasegawa J, Izawa S, Hirakawa Y, Shimokata H, et al. Impact of caregiver burden on adverse health outcomes in community-dwelling dependent older care recipients. American Journal of Geriatric Psychiatry. 2011;**19**(4):382-391

[6] Kazemi A, Azimian J, Mafi M, Allen KA, Motalebi SA. Caregiver burden and coping strategies in caregivers of older patients with stroke. BMC Psychology. 2021;**9**(1):51

[7] Cross AJ, Garip G, Sheffield D. The psychosocial impact of caregiving in dementia and quality of life: A systematic review and meta-synthesis of qualitative research. Psychology and Health. 2018;**33**:1321-1342. DOI: 10.1080/08870446.2018.1496250

[8] Rezaei H, Niksima SH, Ghanei GR. Burden of Care in Caregivers of Iranian patients with chronic disorders: A systematic review and meta-analysis. Health and Quality of Life Outcomes. 2020;**18**(1):261

[9] Arroyo E, Arana A, Garrido R. Crespo R analysis of caregiver burden on dialysis patient. Enfermería Nefrológica. 2018;**21**(3):213-224

[10] Borsje P, Hems MA, Lucassen PL, Bor H, Koopmans RT, Pot AM. Psychological distress in informal caregivers of patients with dementia in primary care: Course and determinants. Family Practice. Aug 2016;**33**(4):374-381

[11] Irianda R, Orizaga C, Chacón P, Chávez V. Impacto de la sobrecarga de los cuidadores de pacientes en diálisis peritoneal. Revista Médica del Instituto Mexicano del Seguro Social. 2020;**58**(2):131-136

[12] Yu Y, Hu J, Efird JT, Mccoy TP. Social support, coping strategies and health-related quality of life among primary caregivers of stroke survivors in China. Journal of Clinical Nursing. 2013;**22**(15-16):2160-2171

[13] Alshammari B, Noble H, McAneney H, Alshammari F, O'Halloran P. Caregiver burden in informal caregivers of patients in Saudi Arabia receiving Hemodialysis: A mixed-methods study. Healthcare (Basel). 2023;**11**(3):1-18

[14] Van Pilsum Rasmussen SE, Eno A, Bowring MG, Lifshitz R,

Garonzik-Wang JM, Al Ammary F, et al. Kidney dyads: Caregiver burden and relationship strain among partners of dialysis and transplant patients. Transplantation Direct. 2020;**6**(7):e566

[15] Vasquez-Jimenez E, Madero M. Global dialysis perspective: Mexico. Kidney. 2020;**360**(1):534-537. DOI: 10.34067/KID.0000912020

[16] Schulz R, Tompkins CA. Informal caregivers in the United States: prevalence, caregiver characteristics, and ability to provide care. In: The Role of Human Factors in Home Health Care. Workshop Summary; 2010. pp. 117-143

[17] Oliver MJ, Abra G, Béchade C, Brown EA, Sanchez-Escuredo A. Assisted peritoneal dialysis: Position paper for the ISPD. Peritoneal Dialysis International. 2024;**44**(3):160-170

[18] Nagasawa H, Sugita I, Tachi T, et al. The relationship between dialysis patients' quality of life and Caregivers' quality of life. Frontiers in Pharmacology. 2018;**9**:770. DOI: 10.3389/fphar.2018.00770

[19] Gilbertson EL, Krishnasamy R, Foote C, et al. Burden of care and quality of life among caregivers for adults receiving maintenance dialysis: A systematic review. American journal of kidney diseases. American Journal of Kidney Diseases. 2019;**73**:332-343. DOI: 10.1053/j.ajkd.2018.09.006

[20] Zarit SH, Reever KE, Bach-Peterson J. Relatives of the impaired elderly: correlates of feelings of burden. Gerontologist. Dec 1980;**20**(6):649-655

[21] Gerritsen JC, van der Ende PC. The development of a care-giving burden scale. Age and Ageing. 1994;**23**(6):483-491. DOI: 10.1093/ageing/23.6.483

[22] Robinson BC. Validation of a caregiver strain index. Journal of Gerontology. 1983;**38**:344-348

[23] Given CW et al. The caregiver reaction assessment (CRA) for caregivers to persons with chronic physical and mental impairments. Research in Nursing and Health. 1992;**15**(4):271-283. DOI: 10.1002/nur.4770150406

[24] Ware JE Jr, Sherbourne CD. The MOS 36-item short-form health survey (SF-36). I. Conceptual framework and item selection. Medical Care. 1992;**30**(6):473-483

[25] Beck AT et al. An inventory for measuring depression. Archives of General Psychiatry. 1961;**4**:561-571. DOI: 10.1001/archpsyc.1961.01710120031004

[26] Teixidó-Planas J, Tarrats Velasco L, Arias Suárez N, Cosculluela MA. Sobrecarga de los cuidadores de pacientes de diálisis peritoneal. Validación de cuestionario y baremos. Nefrología. 2018;**38**(5):459-572. DOI: 10.1016/j.nefro.2018.02.006

[27] Honea NJ, Brintnall R, Given B, Sherwood P, Colao DB, Somers SC, et al. Putting evidence into practice: Nursing assessment and interventions to reduce family caregiver strain and burden. Clinical Journal of Oncology Nursing. Jun 2008;**12**(3):507-516. DOI: 10.1188/08.CJON

[28] Shankar R, Luo N, Lim YW, Khatri P, Leong L, Teo GY, et al. Assessing caregiver burden in advanced kidney disease: Protocol for a systematic review of the measurement properties of instruments and tools. BMJ Open. 2024;**14**(2):e078767. DOI: 10.1136/bmjopen-2023-078767

[29] Oveyssi J, Manera KE, Baumgart A, Cho Y, Forfang D, Saxena A, et al. Patient

and caregiver perspectives on burnout in peritoneal dialysis. Peritoneal Dialysis International. 2021;**41**(5):484-493

[30] Li PK, Chow KM, Cho Y, Fan S, Figueiredo AE, Harris T, et al. ISPD peritonitis guideline recommendations: 2022 update on prevention and treatment. Peritoneal Dialysis International. 2022;**42**(2):110-153

[31] Zhang L, Lee WC, Wu CH, Kuo LC, Yang HT, Moi SH, et al. Importance of non-medical reasons for dropout in patients on peritoneal dialysis. Clinical and Experimental Nephrology. 2020;**24**(11):1050-1057

[32] Lam MF, Leung JC, Lo WK, Tam S, Chong MC, Lui SL, et al. Hyperleptinaemia and chronic inflammation after peritonitis predicts poor nutritional status and mortality in patients on peritoneal dialysis. Nephrology, Dialysis, Transplantation. 2007;**22**(5):1445-1450. DOI: 10.1093/ndt/gfl788

[33] Zalunardo NY, Rose CL, Ma IW, Altmann P. Higher serum C-reactive protein predicts short and long-term outcomes in peritoneal dialysis-associated peritonitis. Kidney International. 2007;**71**(7):687-692. DOI: 10.1038/sj.ki.5002127

[34] Van Diepen AT, van Esch S, Struijk DG, Krediet RT. The first peritonitis episode alters the natural course of peritoneal membrane characteristics in peritoneal dialysis patients. Peritoneal Dialysis International. 2014;**35**(3):324-332. DOI: 10.3747/pdi.2014.00277

[35] Ye H, Zhou Q, Fan L, Guo Q, Mao H, Huang F, et al. The impact of peritoneal dialysis-related peritonitis on mortality in peritoneal dialysis patients. BMC Nephrology. 2017;**18**(1):186

[36] Ye H, Lin X, Qiu Y, Guo Q, Huang F, Yu X, et al. Higher alkaline phosphatase was associated with the short-term adverse outcomes of peritoneal dialysis-related peritonitis. Clinical Chemistry and Laboratory Medicine. 2015;**53**(4):e113-e116

[37] Guedes M, Wallim L, Guetter CR, Jiao Y, Rigodon V, Mysayphonh C, et al. Fatigue in incident peritoneal dialysis and mortality: A real-world side-by-side study in Brazil and the United States. PLoS One. 2022;**17**(6):e0270214. DOI: 10.1371/journal.pone.0270214

[38] Oliver MJ, Salenger P. Making assisted peritoneal dialysis a reality in the United States: A Canadian and American viewpoint. Clinical Journal of the American Society of Nephrology. 2020;**15**(4):566-568

[39] Piarulli P, Vizzardi V, Alberici F, Riva H, Aramini M, Regusci L, et al. Peritoneal dialysis discontinuation: To the root of the problem. Journal of Nephrology. 2023;**36**(7):1763-1776. DOI: 10.1007/s40620-023-01759-w

[40] Oliver MJ, Quinn RR, Richardson EP, Kiss AJ, Lamping DL, Manns BJ. Home care assistance and the utilization of peritoneal dialysis. Kidney International. 2007;**71**(7):673-678

[41] Griva K, Goh CS, Kang WCA, Yu ZL, Chan MC, Wu SY, et al. Quality of life and emotional distress in patients and burden in caregivers: A comparison between assisted peritoneal dialysis and self-care peritoneal dialysis. Quality of Life Research. 2016;**25**(2):373-384

[42] Suri RS, Larive B, Garg AX, Hall YN, Pierratos A, FHN Study Group. Burden on caregivers as perceived by hemodialysis patients in the frequent Hemodialysis network (FHN) trials.

Nephrology, Dialysis, Transplantation. 2011;**26**(7):2316-2322

[43] Rabiei L, Eslami AA, Abbasi M, Afzali SM, Hosseini SM, Masoudi R. Evaluating the effect of family-Centered intervention program on care burden and self-efficacy of Hemodialysis patient caregivers based on social cognitive theory: A randomized clinical trial study. Korean Journal of Family Medicine. 2020;**41**(2):84-90. DOI: 10.4082/kjfm.18.0079

[44] Belasco AG, Sesso R. Burden and quality of life of caregivers for hemodialysis patients. American Journal of Kidney Diseases. 2002;**39**(4):805-812

[45] Hemmati Maslakpak M, Torabi M, Radfar M, Alinejad V. The effect of psycho-educational intervention on the caregiver burden among caregivers of Hemodialysis patients. Journal of Research Development in Nursing and Midwifery. 2019;**16**(1):13-24

Chapter 9

Peritoneal Dialysis in Iraq: Past, Present and Future

Ali Jasim Al Saedi, Nariman Fahmi Ahmed Azat, Yasir Fathi Sharba and Dalia Mahmood Ali

Abstract

The process known as peritoneal dialysis (PD) has become widely accepted in the treatment of both chronic as well as acute kidney injury due to its ease of use and benefits over other forms of dialytic treatment like hemodialysis (HD). As a result, during the past 40 years, PD has been widely used in many large and small hospitals to treat renal injury. PD was first used in September 1967 for a fourteen-year-old patient with acute kidney injury post vibriosis. Since then, acute intermittent peritoneal dialysis (AIPD) has been widely used in different centers all over Iraq. Pediatric patients had shared this practice in pediatric dialysis units as well as adults who usually had contraindications to hemodialysis. Attempts to have continuous ambulatory peritoneal dialysis (CAPD) and automated peritoneal dialysis (APD) were tried in the early 1990s but were not successful because of a lack of access to maintain and sustain solutions and task forces to have a successful insertion of intraperitoneal catheters properly. PD is still an effective treatment for acute kidney damage in children in developing countries, though, particularly in cases where patients have severe coagulation abnormalities, hemodynamic compromise, difficulty gaining vascular access, and a shortage of blood lines suitable for children.

Keywords: peritoneal dialysis, acute kidney injury, acute intermittent, continuous ambulatory, fluids

1. Introduction

Though Nephrology is still considered the most complicated specialty in medicine, it continues to be "The Queen of the Battle". In the globe, chronic kidney disease is scoring the highest among other diseases [1].

Almost 750 million people are suffering from renal diseases because of the increased incidence and prevalence of diabetes mellitus, the leading cause of end-stage kidney disease (ESKD) along with hypertension, obesity, cardiovascular diseases, increased age, glomerular diseases with cystic diseases of the kidney, and other hereditary diseases [2].

Acute kidney injury (AKI) is a major source of morbidity and death in critically ill individuals as well as older people in developing countries. Intra-ICU patients with sepsis, cardiorenal syndrome, and hemodynamic instability make up 30% of the patient population. The dialysis methods utilized in AKI include hemodialysis (HD), continuous renal replacement therapy (CRRT), and acute intermittent peritoneal dialysis (AIPD), which can be performed manually or, in more modern facilities, with an automated system. Since PD is an affordable option for treating AKI, it is frequently utilized in rural locations where access to power, clean water, and water treatment centers is limited. This is particularly true in developing countries, where big cities and towns are the primary locations of renal replacement centers [3].

In this chapter, we discuss how we can maintain peritoneal dialysis to vitally maintain and sustain the service in the face of the horizontal expansion of hemodialysis services where more needs for establishing buildings, more human resources, and continuous electricity are required. Health economy costs from all aspects will save more facilities and effort.

2. History of peritoneal dialysis in Iraq

The first AIPD was attempted in September 1967. A fourteen-year-old patient was admitted to the medical ward in Medical City Hospital, Baghdad, Iraq, because of AKI as a result of severe dehydration post vibriosis. Dr. Thamer Ahmed, a pediatrician who first did AIPD rescued the life of that patient [4, 5].

Renal replacement therapy options for pediatric patients with AKI are numerous and comprise CRRT, HD, and PD [5, 6].

However, the main disadvantages of HD and CRRT therapies are their increasing financial burden and reliance on technology. Because pediatric patients require specialized blood pumps, hemofilters, and blood lines of different sizes to suit both large and small patients, the use of CRRT therapies is even more dependent on technology than it is in adult patients [6, 7].

Furthermore, in order to safely administer these complex techniques, specialized nursing workers with experience caring for such patients are required. When compared to continuous dialysis, AIPD requires significantly fewer financial resources, equipment, and technical know-how [8, 9].

3. Acute intermittent peritoneal dialysis

3.1 Outcome and complications of acute intermittent peritoneal dialysis in Al-Kindi Teaching Hospital

Patients hospitalized in the dialysis unit of Al-Kindi Teaching Hospital underwent AIPD, which was a safe, straightforward procedure that required less skill than HD and had complication rates that were almost identical to those of other reputable centers.

A cross-sectional study on adult patients who had undergone PD and were admitted to the dialysis unit at Al-Kindi Teaching Hospital was conducted between January 2011 and June 2012. In order for staff to assess the etiology of kidney failure, the

	Causes	No.	%
Acute renal failure	Acute tubular necrosis	80	11.96
	Rapidly progressive GN	35	5.23
	Acute interstitial nephritis	32	4.78
	Obstructive uropathy	11	1.64
	Hepatorenal syndrome	10	1.49
	Total	168	25.11
Chronic renal failure	Diabetic nephropathy	170	25.41
	Chronic GN	102	15.25
	Hypertension	94	14.05
	Chronic pyelonephritis	72	10.76
	Obstructive uropathy	63	9.42
	Total	501	74.89
Total		669	100

Source: Al-Saedi [10].

Table 1.
Causes of renal failure of patients.

Indication	No. of patients	%
Metabolic acidosis	214	31.98
Encephalopathy	169	25.26
Fluid overload	151	22.57
Hyperkalemia	82	12.26
Pericarditis	29	4.35
Uremic symptoms	24	3.58
Total	669	100

Source: Al-Saedi [10].

Table 2.
Indications of acute dialysis.

appropriateness of dialysis, the comorbidities, and the prognosis of PD, we created a form (**Tables 1** and **2**).

Of the patients, 349 had complications (52%). Bleeding in the peritoneal cavity was the most frequent problem (30%), followed by a dialysis solution leak (25%). Peritonitis-related complications to dialysis episodes were 2.5%. The death rate was 15% (**Tables 3** and **4**).

In conclusion, Al-Kindi Teaching Hospital successfully and safely carried out AIPD. Tighter nursing precautions and more stringent supervision of new physicians could lead to improvements [10].

	Complications*	Number of episodes	%
Mechanical	Bleeding	201	30
	Peritoneal solution leak	167	25
	Abdominal pain	147	22
	Bowel perforation	1	0.15
Metabolic	Hyperkalemia	132	20
	Hyperglycemia	33	5
Infection	Peritonitis	17	2.5

*Source: Al-Saedi [10]. *The patient may develop more than one complication at the same time.*

Table 3.
Complications of acute intermittent peritoneal dialysis.

<table>
<tr><th rowspan="2">Causes of death</th><th colspan="2">Acute renal failure</th><th colspan="2">Chronic renal failure</th><th rowspan="2">Total no.</th><th rowspan="2">P value</th></tr>
<tr><th>No.</th><th>%</th><th>No.</th><th>%</th></tr>
<tr><td>Septicemia</td><td>33</td><td>49.25</td><td>6</td><td>18.18</td><td>39</td><td>0.005</td></tr>
<tr><td>Brain stem stroke</td><td>20</td><td>29.85</td><td rowspan="2">16</td><td rowspan="2">48.48</td><td>36</td><td>0.11</td></tr>
<tr><td>Acute leukemia</td><td>3</td><td>4.48</td><td>3</td><td>0.54</td></tr>
<tr><td>Myocardial infarction</td><td rowspan="2">8</td><td rowspan="2">11.94</td><td>7</td><td>21.21</td><td>15</td><td>0.36</td></tr>
<tr><td>Pericardial tamponade</td><td rowspan="2">4</td><td rowspan="2">12.12</td><td>4</td><td>0.55</td></tr>
<tr><td>Hepatorenal syndrome</td><td>3</td><td>4.48</td><td>3</td><td>0.54</td></tr>
<tr><td>Total</td><td>67</td><td>100</td><td>33</td><td>100</td><td>100</td><td>0.001</td></tr>
</table>

Source: Al-Saedi [10].

Table 4.
Causes of death in patients on intermittent peritoneal dialysis.

3.2 Peritoneal dialysis in children with acute renal failure in Ibn Al-Balady hospital

This study is a retrospective analysis of 125 children who were admitted to the dialysis unit at the Ibn Al-Balaydy Hospital for Pediatrics and Gynecology between August 2011 and April 2014 (a period of 32 months). Of the 125 children admitted during this period, only 82 patients were included in the analysis; the remaining 34 patients had chronic kidney failure, 15 of whom had incomplete or missing records.

The 82 children in the study had a mean age of 13 + 19.5 months, with 47 (57.3%) of them being male. All patients (100%) had azotemia, with 60 (73.2%) having oliguria, 26 (31.7%) having anuria, 32 (39%), having volume overload, and 28 (32.9%) having encephalopathy. For 32 patients (39%), the most common cause of AKI was sepsis; for 16 patients (19.5%), glomerulonephritis affected 10 individuals (12.2%), and hemolytic uremic syndrome (HUS) affected 9 patients (11%). The most common PD consequence occurring in 33 (40.2%) of patients is peritonitis. Septicemia (63%) and the prevalence of fluid overload, peritonitis, encephalopathy, and anuria (66.7, 66.7, 63, and 59.3%), respectively, were the main causes of the total mortality of 32.9% (**Table 5**).

Variable	Category	Non-survivors (n = 27)
Age	<1 y	23 (85.2)
	>1 y	4 (14.8)
Sex	Male	15 (55.6)
	Female	12 (44.4)
Fluid overload*	Presence	18 (66.7)
	Absence	9 (33.3)
Anuria*	Presence	16 (59.3)
	Absence	11 (40.7)
Encephalopathy*	Presence	17 (63.0)
	Absence	10 (37.0)
Peritonitis*	Presence	18 (66.7)
	Absence	9 (33.3)
Causes	Septicemia*	17 (63.0)
	HUS	5 (18.5)
	Gastroenteritis	2 (7.4)
	GN	1 (3.7)
	Post renal	1 (3.7)

Source: Salim Zyarah Abdullah [11].

Table 5.
Outcome of pediatric patients treated with PD.

In summary, AIPD is the recommended renal replacement therapy option for children experiencing AKI due to its ease of use and practicality, particularly for patients who are hemodynamically unstable and neonates or early infants. The significant death rate in pediatric AKI is attributed to both septicemia and the severity of the condition. Reducing death rates greatly benefits from early identification and referral of individuals who are at risk [11, 12].

3.3 Indications and complications of peritoneal dialysis in children with acute renal failure, a single-center experience

Fifty-nine (59) children with AKI who were admitted to the Child Welfare Teaching Hospital between April 20, 2012 and May 1, 2014, are included in this retrospective investigation.

In the present study, 59 children, ages ranging from 8 days to 15 years, with AKI were enrolled; 23 (39%) were female and 36 (61%) were male. AKI was primarily caused by sepsis (71.1%), hemolytic uremic syndrome (10.9%), and congenital abnormalities of the renal system (13, 22%). Dialysis-related complications were considerably rare among the patients in the study (18.6%; $p < 0.001$). Category dysfunction accounted for 45% of dialysis-related complications. One case of peritonitis (9%; $p = 0.01$). After PD, 42 individuals showed improvement in their renal function. Ninety-seven (6%) of these patients survived ($p < 0.001$). In all, 22% of people died. Severe sepsis accounted for 57% of the patient deaths. Conclusions: AIPD remains a viable and easy-to-achieve treatment option for kids with AKI (**Table 6**) [13].

Variable	Death		Survival		x^2	P
	No.	%	No.	%		
Recovery of renal function						
Yes	1	2.4	41	97.6	32.7*	<0.001
No	12	70.6	5	29.4		
Causes of ARE						
Dehydration	1	25.0	3	75.0	7.8*	0.7
Sepsis	4	57.1	3	42.9		
Hemolytic uremic syndrome	2	20.0	8	80.0		
Glomerulonephritis	0		1	100.0		
Nephrotic syndrome	1	20.0	4	80.0		
Polycystic kidney	0		1	100.0		
Poisoning	0		4	100.0		
metabolic disease	1	20.0	4	80.0		
Congenital malformation of renal system	3	23.1	10	76.9		
SLE nephropathy	0		2	100.0		
Obstructive uropathy	1	33.3	2	66.7		
Acute on chronic renal failure	0		4	100.0		

*Source: Nariman [13]. *Fishers exact test.*

Table 6.
Correlation between recovery of renal function and causes of acute renal failure with outcome of the study group after PD.

4. Continuous ambulatory peritoneal dialysis

Over 750 million people worldwide suffer from the debilitating condition known as chronic kidney disease (CKD), which is impacting roughly 10–15% of the population [14].

4.1 Spectrum of complications of patients with chronic kidney disease on maintenance continuous ambulatory peritoneal dialysis: An experience of tertiary nephrology Center in Najaf City, Iraq

This cross-sectional study included 140 patients (74 women and 66 men) who were receiving dialysis at the renal center for CKD under managed care plans (MCAPD). The participants ranged in age from 18 to 80 years. Participants with PD or HD diagnoses and acute renal disease were not allowed to participate in this study.

There is a notable variation in the distribution of complications by gender in the present study, with female patients having a greater prevalence of both infected and non-infectious issues. The study also found that, as compared to open procedures, the rate of complications among patients undergoing laparoscopic procedures is significantly lower. Furthermore, the problems were more advanced in open abdomen PD patients than in laparoscope maintenance continuous ambulatory peritoneal dialysis (CAPD) patients (**Figure 1**).

In summary, out of all the consequences found in this study, peritoneal infection is the most common. When compared to HD and open surgery, the rate of problems among individuals with PD and laparoscopy is significantly reduced (**Figure 2**) [15, 16].

4.2 Variation of thyroid hormone levels in patients receiving peritoneal dialysis

The kidney plays an important role in thyroid hormone metabolism and iodine excretion. In addition to structural and functional changes in the thyroid gland, malnourishment and increased catabolism are associated conditions in CKD that affect the thyroid's hormone metabolism on their own. In contrast, the Wolff-Chaikoff phenomenon is caused by a decrease in iodine excretion in end-stage renal complications (ERCs), which results in an increase in plasma levels and their inorganic component. Data from uremic patients indicate that iodine's incorporation into thyroid hormones may be reduced.

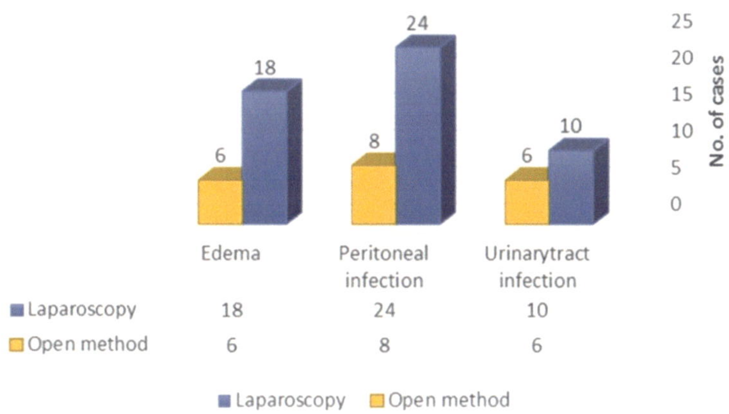

Figure 1.
Distribution of complications according to the type of operation. Source: Sharba [15].

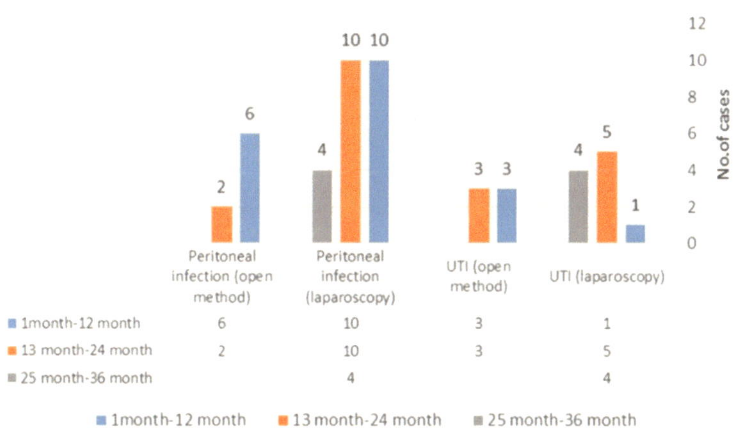

Figure 2.
Distribution of infection according to time of occurrence. Source: Sharba [15].

A total of 100 patients—63 males and 37 women—were examined. The major modality of PD was continuous ambulatory; the average age was 58.2 years, and the average duration of PD was 29.2 ± 3.7 months. Roughly three-quarters of the participants exhibited at least one change in thyroid hormone; 36 of them had subclinical hypothyroidism, while seven had primary hypothyroidism (PH). Conclusions: Thyroid profile screening is a good idea for PD patients [17].

4.3 Outcomes and trends in continuous ambulatory peritoneal dialysis: A retrospective analysis at Najaf Centers (2014–2022)

Retrospective data collection was conducted on patients who began CAPD between 2014 and 2022. Demographic information, method survival, transfers to alternative dialysis modalities, and patient outcomes, including death, were all included in the study. The trends and related complications of the three methods used to introduce CAPD catheters—open laparotomy, percutaneous incision, and laparoscopic—were also examined.

In terms of technique, percutaneous insertions required more revisions and were more likely to result in infection issues than laparoscopic insertions, which demonstrated higher patency rates and fewer early difficulties. Laparoscopic CAPD had the highest technique success rate (79.5%), followed by open laparotomy (46.5%) and percutaneous CAPD (45.6%) (**Figure 3**).

In conclusion, renal replacement therapy such as CAPD is essential, but it is not without risk, including death. To improve patient care and clinical procedures in CAPD, it is imperative to consider the findings of this study on technique efficiency, patient outcomes, and causes of death. The change at Najaf Centers from open laparotomy to laparoscopic treatments is consistent with a larger trend in medicine toward less invasive procedures, which this study has demonstrated to have superior results from [18, 19].

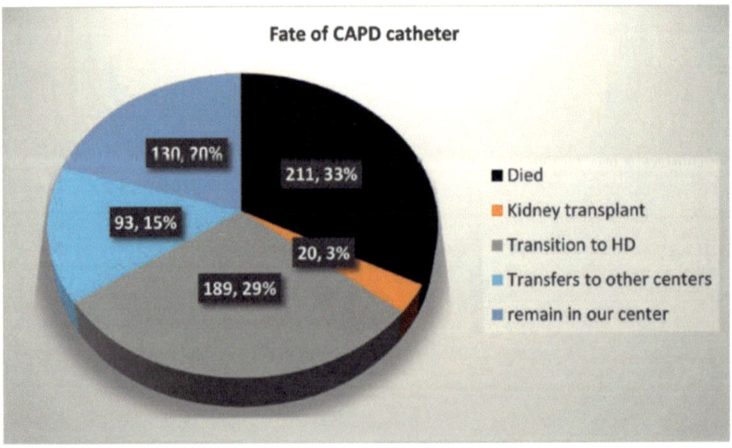

Figure 3.
The fate of CAPD catheter. Source: Sharba [18].

Requirements for inclusion	Criteria for exclusion
Iraqi adults with end-stage renal illnesses who were 18 years of age or older had CAPD	Individuals suffering from cancerous illnesses
A provincial resident of Al-Najaf	Numerous operations on the abdomen
Enrolled at the Middle Euphrates Peritoneal Dialysis Facility	Neglected to follow-up
Men and women in equal measure	Information missing from the medical record

Table 7.
Show the inclusion and exclusion criteria [20].

4.4 Outcomes of continuous ambulatory peritoneal dialysis in treatment of end-stage renal disease in patients registered at Middle Euphrates Center for Peritoneal Dialysis

This cross-sectional study was carried out in the Iraqi province of Al-Najaf, which is situated in the center of the country and roughly 160 kilometers south of Baghdad, the capital. The Middle Euphrates Peritoneal Dialysis Center, a specialized facility under the Najaf Health Directorate, served as the study's location. Data for the cases that were registered and handled by CAPD before 2022 was gathered retrospectively for this study, while prospective data was collected for newly attended cases that were recorded between mid-2023 and mid-2024. The study population comprised all enrolled patients under CAPD management at our facility, from which 93 individuals were chosen as a sample based on the eligibility requirements (inclusion and exclusion standards) shown in **Table 7**.

The "do it yourself" option known as CAPD has emerged as a viable substitute for hospital-based or HD, offering advantages to patients, their families, and the healthcare system. In several centers throughout Iraq, the majority of patients continue to receive their dialysis in hospitals, and CAPD is not commonly used there. In the present study, we evaluated the effects of CAPD in end-stage renal disease patients enrolled at the Middle Euphrates Peritoneal Dialysis Center in Najaf City.

CAPD, a "do it yourself" option that benefits individuals, their households, and the health care system, has become a competitive alternative to hospital-based or home HD. The majority of patients in a number of sites across Iraq still receive their dialysis in hospitals, and CAPD is not frequently utilized there. In the present study, individuals with end-stage renal illness who were recruited at the Middle Euphrates Peritoneal Dialysis Center in Najaf City were tested for the effects of CAPD [21].

5. Current and planned PD program in Iraq

There is a tremendous increase in both prevalence and incidence of CKD in the country, with 14% of the Iraqi population (45.6 million) having CKD. One million and 600.000 are having CKD (grades 3–5). The number of HD centers has been increasingly expanded from 40 to 120 centers to face challenges. The vision is to create highly effective PD facilities to recruit 20–30% of patients who have CAPD or APD.

The presence of proper infrastructure as regard centers devoted to PD in different governments in Iraq, including well-established centers in Najaf in the middle of Iraq and Basra in the south, with a big training and educational center in Medical City, the biggest teaching center in Iraq, as well as in Mousel, north of Iraq. With the presence of a highly trained PD medical staff dedicated to PD service, the service will be set for success. A highly skilled surgical team to insert PD catheters is already available with accumulative experience in the field.

The giant step was to have a contract to manufacture all types of PD fluids in Iraq under MOH supervision—a step to maintain the availability of fluids and to sustain supply to patients in the long run.

Acute dialysis was indicated for metabolic acidosis, uremic symptoms, fluid overload, hyperkalemia, pericarditis, and uremic encephalopathy.

PD complications were categorized as mechanical, metabolic, and infectious. There were 349 individuals with problems, representing a 52% risk of occurrence.

One hundred people lost their lives. Thirty-three patients remained with chronic renal failure, while 67 patients died of acute renal failure. Since PD patients had well-controlled plasma biochemistry, the underlying illness—rather than uremia—was the cause of death. Uremia is directly responsible for only four of the deaths.

The degree of renal failure has a major impact on the prognosis of peritoneal dialysis (PD). Of the 35 patients who presented with fluid overload, 20 died during or shortly after PD, accounting for 74.1% of deaths; the 17 patients who died from encephalopathy accounted for 63% of deaths. Patients receiving PD treatment were at significantly higher risk of dying from septicemia and peritonitis (as a consequence of either septicemia or PD) (p value <0.05). Out of the 32 patients diagnosed with septicemia, 17 of them died (63% of deaths), while 18 of the patients diagnosed with peritonitis (66.7%) also died.

Renal function recovery and outcome were statistically significantly correlated ($p < 0.001$). In patients whose renal function did not return, about two-thirds of them died.

Figure 1 shows the distribution of complications according to the type of operation used in CAPD either open method or laparoscopy.

Figure 2 shows the distribution of infections by the time of incidence following CAPD, either by laparoscopy or open technique.

Of these, 432 patients had either switched to another modality or were still on CAPD; 211 of the patients had died. In our facility, 130 patients with CAPD remained to have a decent quality of life, 189 were switched to hemodialysis, and 20 patients underwent kidney transplants. The government newly created facilities will provide funding for the remaining 93 transfers.

6. Conclusions

Using PD as their "initial" renal replacement therapy (RRT) modality would probably help more patients due to its greater survival in the first 2 years. Strong arguments for starting PD include schedule flexibility, the potential to avoid necessary hospital visits, which saves time, and the simplicity of doing dialysis at home. Patients with peritoneal dialysis are not limited in any way in their travel, employment, or social activities. While infections among HD patients have increased, PD-related infections have decreased as a result of technique developments. Thus, there is a higher chance of septicemia, hospitalization, and death for HD patients.

For prospective receivers, PD is the preferred modality because transplant patients with prior PD are more likely to have a faster reduction in plasma creatinine, be less likely to develop delayed graft function and have a lower chance of transplant failure or death. PD usually permits the initial preservation of residual renal function (RRF) in the majority of patients because of the native kidneys' contribution to improved intermediate molecular clearance, fluid status, heart function, nutrition, hemoglobin levels, bone mineral metabolism, and overall standard of living.

Acknowledgements

To all colleagues who spent days and nights offering services whether AIPD, CAPD in Baghdad, Mousel, Basra, Nassirya, Najaf Furat Ausat Center for Peritoneal Dialysis. Trying their best to rescue lives of infants and adults and prolong their survival.

Conflict of interest

The authors declare no conflict of interest.

Acronyms and abbreviations

AIPD	acute intermittent peritoneal dialysis
CAPD	continuous ambulatory peritoneal dialysis
AKI	acute kidney injury
CKD	chronic kidney disease
HD	hemodialysis
CRRT	continuous renal replacement therapy

Author details

Ali Jasim Al Saedi[1*], Nariman Fahmi Ahmed Azat[2*], Yasir Fathi Sharba[3*] and Dalia Mahmood Ali[4*]

1 College of Medicine, University of Baghdad, Nephrology and Renal Transplantation Center, Baghdad, Iraq

2 College of Medicine, Baghdad University, Iraq

3 Al_Furat Al_Aosat Center for Peritoneal Dialysis and Alnajaf Teaching Hospital, Alnajaf, Iraq

4 Child Welfare Teaching Hospital, Medical City, Baghdad, Iraq

*Address all correspondence to: alsaedinephrology@gmail.com; ali.alsaedy@meciq.edu.com, narimanfahmi@comed.uobaghdad.edu.iq, yasirsharba1971@gmail.com and dr.dalia8181@yahoo.com

References

[1] Matthews DE, West KW, Rescorla FJ, Vane DW, Grosfeld JL, Wappner RS, et al. Peritoneal dialysis in the first 60 days of life. Journal of Pediatric Surgery. 1990;**25**:110-116

[2] Pedersen KR, Hjortdal VE, Christensen S, Pedersen J, Hjortholm K, Larsen SH, et al. Clinical outcome in children with acute renal failure treated with peritoneal dialysis after surgery for congenital heart disease. Kidney International. Supplement. 2008;**108**:S81-S86

[3] Abraham G, Varughese S, Mathew M, Vijayan M. A review of acute and chronic peritoneal dialysis in developing countries. Clinical Kidney Journal. 2015;**8**:310-317

[4] Morelli S, Ricci Z, Di Chiara L, Stazi GV, Polito A, Vitale V, et al. Renal replacement therapy in neonates with congenital heart disease. Contributions to Nephrology. 2007;**156**:428-433

[5] Karkar A, Wilkiehttps M. Peritoneal dialysis in the modern era. Peritoneal Dialysis International. 2023;**43**(4):301-314

[6] Kumar V, Ramachandran R, Rathi M, Kohli HS, Sakhuja V, Jha V. Peritoneal dialysis: The great savior during disasters. Peritoneal Dialysis International. 2013;**33**:327-329

[7] Anochie IC, Eke FU. Acute renal failure in Nigerian children: Port Harcourt experience. Pediatric Nephrology. 2005;**20**:1610-1614

[8] Mishra OP, Gupta AK, Pooniya V, Prasad R, Tiwary NK, Schaefer F. Peritoneal dialysis in children with acute kidney injury: A developing country experience. Peritoneal Dialysis International. 2012;**32**:431-436

[9] Hoste EA, Clermont G, Kersten A, et al. RIFLE criteria for acute kidney injury are associated with hospital mortality in critically ill patients: A cohort analysis. Critical Care. 2006;**10**:R73

[10] Al-Saedi A, J. Outcome and complications of acute intermittent peritoneal dialysis in Al-Kindi teaching hospital. Iraqi Journal of Medical Sciences. 2013;**11**(3):205-210

[11] Abdullah SZ. Peritoneal dialysis in children with acute renal failure in Ibn Al Balady Hospital. The Iraqi Postgraduate Medical Journal Peritoneal Dialysis. 2015;**14**(1):1-6

[12] Burdmann EA, Chakravarthi R. Peritoneal dialysis in acute kidney injury: Lessons learned and applied. Seminars in Dialysis. 2011;**24**:149-156

[13] Azat NFA. Indications and complications of peritoneal dialysis in children with acute renal failure, a single center experience. Journal of the Faculty of Medicine Baghdad. 2016;**58**(2):126-131

[14] Li PK, Chow KM, Van de Luijtgaarden MW, Johnson DW, Jager KJ, Mehrotra R, et al. Changes in the worldwide epidemiology of peritoneal dialysis. Nature Reviews. Nephrology. 2017;**13**(2):90-103. DOI: 10.1038/nrneph.2016.181

[15] Noori E, Hadi R, Sharba Y, Sharba ZF. Spectrum of complications of patients with chronic kidney disease on maintenance continuous ambulatory peritoneal dialysis: An experience of tertiary nephrology

Center in Najaf City-Iraq. Open Access Macedonian Journal of Medical Sciences. 2021;**9**(B):1529-1534

[16] Ataş DB, Aşıcıoğlu E, Tuğcu M, Arıkan İH, Velioğlu A. Long-term predictors of mortality in peritoneal dialysis patients. Turkish Journal of Nephrology. 2021;**30**(3):1-6

[17] Al-Isawi MAA-MI, Almatwari MAM. Variation of thyroid hormone levels in patients receiving peritoneal dialysis. International Journal of Biological Sciences. 2019;**2**(1):82-91

[18] Laith Fathi S, Yasir Fathi S, Mahmood Shaker J, Nazar J. Outcomes and trends in continuous ambulatory peritoneal dialysis: A retrospective analysis at Najaf Centers (2014-2022). Romanian Journal of Medical Practice. 2024;**19**(1):58-63

[19] Chaudhary K, Sangha H, Khanna R. Peritoneal dialysis first: Rationale. Clinical Journal of the American Society of Nephrology. 2011;**6**:447-456

[20] Sharba YFF, Almatwari MAM, NaserHussein Z, Joodi AN. Outcomes of continuous ambulatory peritoneal dialysis in treatment of end stage renal disease in patients registered at middle euphrates center for peritoneal dialysis. AJCS; 2024;**6**(3):142-158

[21] Mansour N, Khalleefah M, Soliman N, Shaglabow S, Abdulgadir S, Ramdan A. Association of Gender, age, physiological, and biochemical parameters among chronic renal failure patients at Zawia Kidney Hospital. Khalij-Libya Journal of Dental and Medical Research. 2023;**7**(2):171-177